MW00990730

I'M DR. RED DUKE

Publication of this book is supported
by a gift from Bob Walker '58,
in memory and honor of his dear wife,
JOANN NOLEN WALKER '92.
She instilled the love of reading in four Aggie children:
Rebecca '81, Sid '82, Richard '86, and Bill '88.
Texas A&M University Press will always hold a special place
in the hearts of the Walker family.

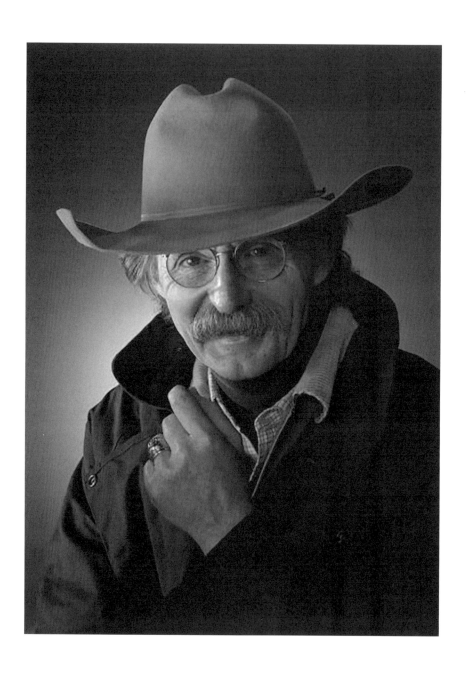

I'M DR. RED DUKE

Bryant Boutwell

Foreword by George H. W. Bush

Texas A&M University Press • College Station

This paper meets the requirements
of ANSI/NISO Z39.48–1992 (Permanence of Paper).
Binding materials have been chosen for durability.
Manufactured in the United States of America

Library of Congress Cataloging-in-Publication Data

Names: Boutwell, Bryant, author. | Bush, George, 1924– writer of foreword.
Title: I'm Dr. Red Duke / Bryant Boutwell; foreword by George H. W. Bush.
Description: First edition. | College Station: Texas A&M University Press,
    [2018] | Includes index.
Identifiers: LCCN 2018013989 | ISBN 9781623496944 (cloth: alk. paper)
Subjects: LCSH: Duke, James H., Jr. (James Henry), 1928–2015. |
    Surgeons—Texas—Houston—Biography. | Medical teaching
    personnel—Texas—Houston—Biography. | Television personalities—United
    States—Biography.
Classification: LCC R154.D85 B68 2018 | DDC 617.092 [B]—dc23 LC record avail-
able at https://lccn.loc.gov/2018013989

For Betty, Patricia, Hank, Rebecca, Sara & Hallie

Contents

Foreword

As a proud Houstonian, I am rather biased about my hometown of some sixty years now. We live in one of the world's great cities, not necessarily because of scenic, sweeping mountain vistas—or perpetually idyllic weather. Rather, it is the can-do spirit of the remarkable people who call this place home that makes Houston so unique, so special.

If you stop to think about it, what other city would—or could—dig a ship channel fifty miles inland? Houstonians are not only dreamers, but also doers. People who think big, and often risk it all daring to follow through. People like Captain Baker and Jesse Jones. Hugh Roy Cullen, Michel Halbouty, and Red Adair, Denton Cooley, and Michael DeBakey.

In my view, no list of the iconic Houstonians who helped build our city, and certainly the Texas Medical Center, is complete without Dr. James Henry "Red" Duke. Red was a Texas original, driven in everything he did by a sense of vocation. Everywhere he went—from Texas A&M to Afghanistan to TV and his respected wildlife conservation work—he was always a leader, always breaking new ground.

Of course, it was Red's pioneering efforts to launch the Life Flight air ambulance service that helped galvanize the Texas Medical Center's status among the world's great trauma care centers. How many thousands of lives have been saved because of his vision and devotion to his patients?

The fact is, we can never repay Red for all he did for our community, but happily, through this terrific book, we can mark his singular achievements—continuing both to learn and to draw inspiration from him.

After all, he reflected the essential Houston spirit. He was humble, driven to help others and to leave this a better world than he found it. In that sense, he was one of the brightest Points of Light Barbara and I have had the privilege to know.

George H. W. Bush

Acknowledgments

For this writer, the research and writing phases of a book are a welcome journey accented by straightaways, unexpected turns, pleasant surprises, and a few dark corners. This book had it all, and I'm thankful to have made the trip. My thanks to Red Duke's wife Betty and her now grown children, Hank, Rebecca, Sara, and Hallie, for guiding me along the way and entrusting me to tell the stories of Red Duke's life. Although Betty remarried (as did Red), she plans to one day be buried in the Texas State Cemetery in Austin next to him and with her Cowden family. I will forever be grateful that during my research Betty opened her home and her stashes of letters and photographs from the early 1950s to shine a bright light on the young seminary student she had married so many years before.

Special thanks are also due to Red's daughter Sara and her husband, Charles King, who admitted me to their home for many a country breakfast with Red. During that first visit, as Red stirred his coffee he wasted no time adding his own acknowledgment to her: "Thank God for Sara and all her family, who've put up with this old fool." Likewise they put up with my frequent visits and unending questions.

Thanks to Sara I found my way into Red's dimly lit storage units, one of the unexpected byways of this journey, where a treasure trove of letters opened up his daily life in decades past. Less than a month after his death, I found myself again with Sara and Charles in Red's medical school office, where late into the evening we boxed his possessions. Every inch was buried deep in papers and keepsakes, an archeological dig that gave up otherwise irretrievable information about his life.

Betty and I went on a road trip back to Hillsboro so that I could meet Red's sister, Patricia. In a busy Mexican food restaurant just a stone's throw from Hillsboro's outlet mall, on a tract of land where Red once picked cotton, Patricia schooled me in Duke family lore. Her memories included a little dog Red pulled out of his football jacket one Christmas morning so long ago. He was named Taps, and according to Patricia,

"Taps fathered puppies all over Hillsboro for years thereafter." There were tears of laughter that afternoon mixed with tears of loss. We drove to the old family home, where Red had addressed so many letters over the years. A pickup truck was parked in the drive. The young family that lives there now knows nothing of the stories the walls could tell.

At the Texas Medical Center I want to thank UTHealth's president, Dr. Giuseppe Colasurdo, who put his confidence in me to take on this project and do justice to the man and the institution. UTHealth is the University of Texas Health Science Center at Houston, Red's home and the scene of so many health reports over the years. It is a big place with a big mission and has an outstanding hospital affiliate, Memorial Hermann–Texas Medical Center. The hospital, which was formerly known simply as Hermann Hospital, is among the best in the nation and is partner not only to UTHealth but also to the McGovern Medical School, where Red found a home in 1972 and never left.

I want to thank President George H. W. Bush, who without reservation agreed to write the foreword for this book to honor his friend. It was a pleasure working with his Houston-based staff.

At UTHealth, Meredith Raine in media relations worked with Red and the family to ensure that throughout his illness and after his death, media and publications would be handled with due care. Karen Kaplan, a friend with oversight of UTHealth communication programs for many years, provided encouragement for early versions of the manuscript. Sheryl Barrett gave the final manuscript a careful review with the eye of a devoted Texas A&M former student. I thank my friend Dr. William Kellar for sharing his Red Duke interview transcripts from past projects. And I thank Dr. Carmel Dyer, Joanie Hernandez-McClain, Heidimarie Porter, and Pamela Kennedy at UTHealth for their encouragement and for listening to my Red Duke stories around the office as I framed the structure for this book.

At the McGovern Medical School, Darla Brown and Dwight Andrews in the Office of Communications opened their photo files for images, as did Phil Montgomery at the McGovern Historical Archives and Research Center, which is part of the Texas Medical Center Library. At the UT Southwestern Medical Center Health Sciences Digital Library and Learning Center in Dallas, my thanks to Cameron Kainerstorfer and Catherine Miller. Also, thanks to the Baylor University Texas Collection and University Archives in Waco, Texas.

I owe special gratitude to my late mentor, Dr. John P. McGovern, whose name now distinguishes our medical school. McGovern loved a good story. He stressed the value of humanism in medicine and the importance of knowing the history behind every story. Not a day goes by since his death in 2007 that I don't hear his voice in my ear.

To the many people I interviewed during the research phase of this project and who appear on these pages, I extend my appreciation. I owe special praise for Margret Kerbaugh, an extraordinary book editor whom I've worked with before. Sometimes the straightaways are not so straight, and a writer gets lost on the turns. Margret is a person who will straighten the wheel instinctively. While she lives far from Texas, in Illinois, she instantly knew the name Red Duke when I approached her about this project, and joined the journey without reservation. For all who read drafts and provided comments and corrections, I am in your debt.

I also want to thank Dr. James Bertz, a multitalented plastic surgeon/dentist who travels the world in retirement helping people who would otherwise not be helped. He spoke at Red's memorial service and enlightened us all, as did Jayar Daily. I met Jayar, a community-minded Houstonian and conservationist, one morning in College Station. Jayar insisted I read several books on conservation if I was to write a word about conservation and Red Duke. He then sent me a list and followed up on my progress. It is a serious topic, and Jayar was serious. I read them all.

For all those at UTHealth and Memorial Hermann–Texas Medical Center who worked beside Red over the years, including his beloved Memorial Hermann Life Flight team, thank you for all you do each and every day. For not a day goes by that a Life Flight helicopter doesn't lift off in a race with the golden hour, with Red's call sign and spirit on board.

And finally, I'd like to express my appreciation for my wife, Lana, and my teenage daughter at home, Mae. Mae attended the dedication of the Red Duke Elementary School in 2014 and dutifully posed for a photo with Red at her parents' request. She was more than self-conscious sitting in the spotlight surrounded by cameras. Sensing her discomfort, Red whispered in her ear words audible only to her. I could only imagine what wisdom Dr. Red Duke imparted that day. He was a great communicator who could connect with any audience, and I anticipated prophetic insights to last her a lifetime. After several days I had to ask.

"He said, 'Don't you just hate it when your parents make you do something you don't want to?'"

I suspect she will always remember the straight-talking doctor she met that day. He won her over instantly—as he has done with so very many others over so very many years.

I'M DR. RED DUKE

Introduction

With his wire-rimmed glasses, bushy mustache, cowboy hat, and unmistakable country drawl, Red Duke was a one-of-a kind, made-in-Texas original. To meet him was to meet the Marlboro Man, Albert Schweitzer, and Teddy Roosevelt all in one—with a good dash of Wile E. Coyote stirred into the mix just for cussedness.

Professionally, Duke combined the commonsense virtues of a small-town country doctor with the skills of a big-city trauma surgeon. But although he was a gifted surgeon, he was many other things as well—a distinguished Eagle Scout, an ordained Baptist minister, a medical missionary to Afghanistan, a builder of trendsetting medical programs (including Memorial Hermann Life Flight, the first air ambulance service in Texas), a conservationist, an Alaskan hunting guide, an army tank commander, a television personality whose health reports were syndicated worldwide, a husband, a father, and a patriot. He was a citizen of this planet with a reverence for life and an inexhaustible knack for living it.

This book is the story of James Henry "Red" Duke Jr., MD, scion of Ennis, Texas—just a cow-patty toss from Dallas, as he would say. He arrived at Houston's Texas Medical Center at the age of forty-four to join the surgical department of the University of Texas Medical School, one of six professional schools composing the University of Texas Health Science Center at Houston—UTHealth, for short.[1] Next door at the medical school's primary affiliate, Hermann Hospital (now known as Memorial Hermann–Texas Medical Center), Red Duke was a name everyone would soon know. The year was 1972, and the medical school was just two years old and still finding its feet. The Houston medical center was rising quickly as one of the largest and best in the nation, and Red Duke wasted no time adding to its momentum.

I arrived in 1974 as a writer for the University of Texas M. D. Anderson Cancer Center. The skies were quiet when I moved into my office. But within two years, helicopters were buzzing over my building like bees over a hive. That sound was made by Life Flight, a new air ambulance program over at Hermann Hospital started by a surgeon named Red Duke.

Within a few years Red Duke was on my television screen every night delivering short, folksy, commonsense health messages completely unlike any I had ever seen or heard before. His sign-off for each segment was delivered with an unmistakable and unforgettable Texas twang: "From the University of Texas Health Science Center at Houston . . . [pause for effect] I'm Dr. Red Duke."

There was clearly a new doc in town, and big names in Houston's Texas Medical Center, like Michael DeBakey (Baylor College of Medicine), Denton Cooley (Texas Heart Institute), and Lee Clark (M. D. Anderson Cancer Center) had better move over.

Fast-forward to 1993, and I'm the associate dean for community affairs and professional education at the UT Medical School at Houston (recently renamed the McGovern Medical School, part of UTHealth). Given my writing and public health background and Red's now far-reaching television enterprise, we were naturally drawn together. It was not unusual to find him at my door straight out of a long night of surgery, wearing a pair of greens that looked slept in and a crinkled white coat that flapped around his long, skinny legs.

Anything might come out of these morning apparitions. On one occasion he strolled past me through the door, swallowing coffee, and said, "Hey, bud. Let's start a health column in Texas Monthly."

I was a little exasperated, because I had not yet had the benefit of coffee, and I may have been slightly annoyed that Duke thought he could just sail into the halls of the mighty *Texas Monthly* and sail out again in possession of a column.

"I'll provide the content and you provide the polish."

"Red," I said, "do you even know anybody at *Texas Monthly?*"

He locked eyes with me, glided into a nearby chair, grabbed my phone, and punched numbers into it out of the air. In seconds he had Mike Levy, founder and publisher of *Texas Monthly*, on the line. Their greetings on speaker phone, followed by chummy talk about camp-outs and barbecue cook-offs, made it clear that I should never assume Red Duke didn't have contacts. Then he got down to business and made his case for the column. "We need to preach some prevention," he said.

"Folks have just gotta realize that most all accidents are preventable. They're living in de-nial, *and that ain't no river in Egypt.*"

The line was cribbed, but Red Duke was a classic. In my four decades of working among the best and brightest physicians and medical educators in the world, I have never again met his kind, and I never expect to, either. But who really was this brilliant, universally loved eccentric with the talented surgical hands and brain and the immense comic-book mustache? Who were his parents, and how did they affect the path he followed? Who were the personal heroes who guided his choices in life and helped set his moral compass? What was behind his indefatigable drive to help other people? "Lord knows I'm not perfect," he was often heard to say. I am a willing believer in Red Duke's imperfections—but what, exactly, were they?

And what about his four children? And his wife of thirty-one years, Betty? They had divorced in 1984. Surely Red Duke's imperfections had more than a little to do with that. But during the last year of his life, Betty and Duke underwent a reunion of heart and head, and Betty was with him to the end. From my vantage point that last year, I saw a love story respooling.

In reality, I never expected to write this book. In what I took for the normal course of events, it would not have been possible to collect the stories of a trauma surgeon as busy as Red Duke, who knew no day or night and never slowed down beyond a quick sprint. But that all changed on the night of April 8, 2013. After a dinner with friends at a Houston restaurant, Duke was taken down by what he would later dismissively term a "pesky heart valve" that had him "all stoved up and out of action." The truth is that he survived the night only through the surgical intervention of his colleagues. But he would never return to the operating room as a surgeon.

Later that week I picked up my phone to hear the news that was about to rock the whole medical school. Red Duke, the grand old man of Memorial Hermann, who had saved thousands of lives and trained the best of the best to go out into the world and do likewise, was now himself a patient in peril of his life.

In time, Duke would pack up a handful of surgical scrubs and allow himself to be moved to his daughter Sara's comfortable house near College Station, about a hundred miles from Houston. Here he would convalesce, and here the faithful would flock, bringing with them the spark of the busy outside world and carrying away Duke's take on it all—and his stories. Here on Saturday mornings I would find him in his wheelchair, making part of the family circle around Sara's breakfast table. It would be steaming with cups of fresh-brewed coffee and sunny with new eggs from the henhouse.[2] And here an idea took shape in my mind.

I decided to pitch a book to him.

"No one wants to read a book about me," he scoffed—disingenuously, of course, because the last forty years of his life had to have taught him better. People were fascinated by him. He had after all gotten to sit down every week for a year and watch a television drama about himself.[3] But humility and self-deprecation were a reflexive part of the persona he had cultivated with wily relish and marked success for decades.

So, perched in a familiar spot somewhere along the continuum between graciousness and irascibility, he submitted. And over the next year, the last year of his life, he allowed me to record long hours of his conversation and reminiscences.

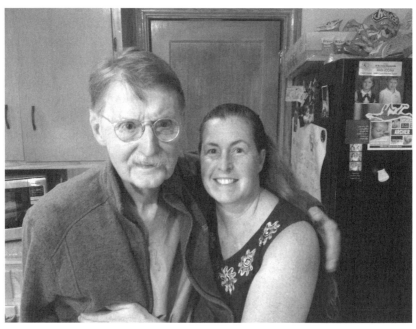

Red and daughter Sara in her kitchen, 2014.

Having a weekend cabin on a lake not a half-hour drive from Sara's house in College Station made it easy for me to call on Saturday mornings. Every visit started at the kitchen table with Sara's country breakfast. Her husband, Charles, was there too, an affable host. And I was the privileged listener to the stories spun by Red Duke, a master storyteller who was never short on either matter or opinion. An oxygen tank supplemented his failing physical strength. But his wit was sharp and his memories of bygone times were readily accessible. His ability to recall detail was extraordinary. He could sketch a surgical technique on a paper napkin without missing a beat of the story he was telling. On Sundays, as I returned from my cabin to Houston, I sometimes stopped again and delivered him catfish filets from the weekend's fishing trip. Stories for catfish—it was pure Red Duke.

Finding a balance between caring for patients around the clock and making time for children and family is never easy for medical doctors, especially trauma surgeons. Some get it right; others struggle and even give up trying. As I sat before Red Duke's coffin during his Houston

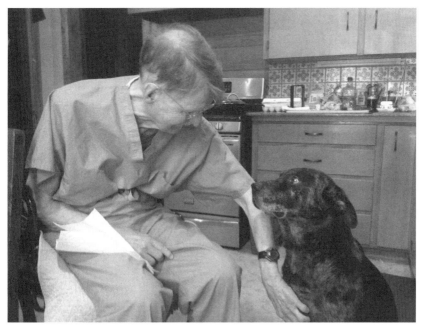

Red and his beloved Jake during a country breakfast visit in 2014.

memorial service for invited family and friends on a hot, sunny August morning in 2015, I could not help looking to my right to see Betty and the four grown children, Hank, Rebecca, Sara, and Hallie. Sara's husband held the leash for Red's dog, Jake, who sat patiently just feet from the flag-draped coffin, looking for his missing master. Red loved that dog. As university officials and former patients droned on with their long and earnest testimony to Red's many contributions to health care, it was clear to me that the family was more than a little lost in the conversation. They didn't know all of the eulogists, and probably much of what these strangers were saying was hard to connect with the man they had known at home. Then, on short notice, everyone in the crowded sanctuary was asked to step outside and await a fly-by of Life Flight helicopters saluting their creator and medical director. Back inside, more tributes followed from colleagues representing Red's medical career and his passion for wildlife conservation.

The man being eulogized was perfect. The man Betty had been married to was more nuanced. She had carried the load of bringing up their children so that he could devote his time and energy to medicine. She and her children had sacrificed important parts—irreplaceable parts— of their lives and identities to share him with the rest of the world. Some of their sacrifices had been made more willingly than others—even on Christmas mornings, the family had to hurry their private exchange of presents before the medical students, residents, and fellows who could not get home for Christmas would start arriving. Red's tendency was always to reach to the outside world first. As they sat at the memorial service, his wife and children knew that he had loved them, and loved them well. But they also knew that they had not come first.

Hours after the memorial service was over and the Life Flight helicopters had returned to their base, the family drove to Austin for a private burial at the Texas State Cemetery.[4] Here Red Duke is at home, surrounded by men and women who, like him, commanded the headlines of their day: governors, statesmen, leaders of many stamps—the heroes of Texas' rich history.

But the sentiment on Red's tombstone sets it apart from the others, which tend to run to the high-toned and platitudinous. Red's is the tombstone of a maverick who did not resort to platitude, even in the

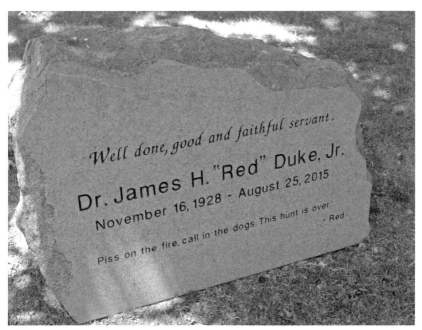

Red's gravestone, Texas State Cemetery, Austin, Texas.

face of mortality. To the dismay of some and the delight of others, it reads, down at the bottom and in small, sly letters:

Piss on the fire, call in the dogs. This hunt is over.

My friend, your hunts may be over, but your memory and your legacy live on.

These, then, are the stories of your life and times.

CHAPTER I
Beginnings

A lot was going on in the world in 1928, the year Red Duke was born. Walt Disney released his first two cartoons with sound. One of them, *Steamboat Willie*, introduced Mickey Mouse to the world. Over in Santa Barbara, a fellow built the first factory making yo-yos. The toy, dating back to 500 BC in China (or Greece, depending on who is telling the story), would be mass produced and become a national sensation. The Roaring Twenties were winding down, but Prohibition was still going strong and Eliot Ness was leading it in Chicago. And in Hollywood, Gary Cooper, a new face on the screen, starred in a World War I silent movie called *Wings*. The movie would win a new award introduced that year, known as the Oscar.

On the medical front, Alexander Fleming was hard at work figuring out a mysterious mold that somehow slipped into his research laboratory and was killing off bacteria in petri dishes he had failed to close. Two years later he would announce his discovery as penicillin. Also during 1928, the iron lung was invented, and Richard Byrd started his famous trek to Antarctica. Calvin Coolidge was president, and in March of 1928 he bestowed the congressional Medal of Honor on Charles Lindberg for his famed transatlantic flight the year before.

In Texas, just an hour and twenty-one minutes past the cold midnight of November 16, in the small railroad town of Ennis, James Henry "Red" Duke Jr. was born. His early-morning arrival did not attract the same attention as the other events we have cited, but in the eighty-six years to come, Red Duke would make his own distinctive mark on the world. In his old age, Duke would look back on his arrival that cold night and observe that things very nearly went awry.

"It was just a little tiny hospital and there certainly were no accreditation standards, computers, or anything like that, and another little fellow was born that night. As I understand it, they took the other little fellow to the lady that I called 'Mother,' so I presume they took me to the other one and I guess I got rejected or something."[1]

But even when he had been safely stowed in the arms of his rightful mother, twenty-seven-year-old Helen Donegan Duke, the confusion was not over. The doctor asked for the baby's name. Helen and her husband, James Henry Duke, two years Helen's senior, hadn't really thought that part through. These devout Baptists were worn down from the events of the early morning and were easy to please. When the Biblical name David came randomly to mind, they took it. "David" Red Duke would be, and the name was duly recorded.

Once home, "My dad took me to town and they would say, 'Oh, you've got a junior,' so he starts calling me James—James Henry Duke Jr. When I went to get my driver's license at age sixteen, I found out I wasn't James, I was David. So, I am not really sure who the hell I am or where I came from."[2]

Word of the new Duke spread quickly around the small town and beyond. Just days after his arrival, Helen's maternal grandmother acknowledged the event in a congratulatory letter from Los Angeles, in which she reported family assurances that the baby "is very handsome and looks like his daddy" and admonished the latter "not to strut too much."[3]

In short order the growing child would develop a headful of bushy red hair, and he would forever be known as "Red," Red Duke. To say Helen doted on him would be an understatement. Despite the difficulties of making a living in Ennis during the early years of the Depression, with the local and national economies plunging, Helen could be seen all over town carrying her infant son, who was tricked out as elaborately as a little prince, as if in defiance of the hard times. In one family photo, a six-year-old Red stands in the yard dressed in a classic Fauntleroy suit with cutaway jacket, matching knee pants, and a short white tie emerging from the rounded collar of his white shirt.

At the time, Helen could hardly appreciate the irony of imposing such sartorial splendor on Red, who, when he had a choice, would drive a battered pickup truck and wear blue jeans and mud-caked cowboy boots.

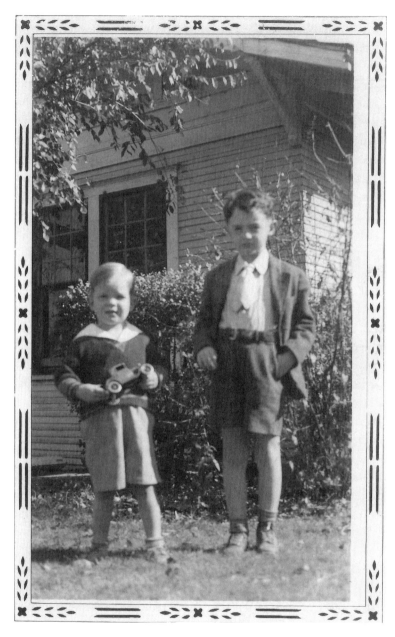

Red (on the right) at age six, well-dressed in a Fauntleroy suit with a neighborhood friend.

Ennis, located in Ellis County, was cotton country. The Blackland Prairie south of Dallas was the heart of the cotton belt, famous for rich, fertile soil with an unlimited capacity for growing cotton. Area farmers noted proudly that samples of Blackland Prairie soil had been collected by the Department of Agriculture in Washington, DC, to determine what mysteries it held to produce such high yields. In the 1880s Texas cultivated up to one-fourth of the world's total cotton crop. Ellis County (its county seat at Waxahachie) boomed after the Civil War. It saw a 600 percent increase in cotton production during just one decade in the late 1800s.[4]

With cotton production from the many small tenant farms that dotted the rural landscape came compresses, oil mills, and numerous other cotton-related industries. When the Houston and Texas Central Railroad (later to become part of the expansive Southern Pacific Railroad) extended its line through eastern Ellis County in 1871, local residents had rail service for the first time. Ennis would become a major rail connecting Dallas to the port cities—a perfect artery of transportation from the cotton fields to Houston and Galveston. In the 1920s, the decade of Red Duke's birth, Dallas became the world's largest producer of cotton gin equipment, with more than half of the gin machinery manufactured right up the road from the Black Prairie soil of Ennis.[5]

On the other end of the rail line, in Houston, were the world's largest cotton merchandizing companies, like Anderson, Clayton and Company, which had the warehouses and international banking and transportation networks to meet the worldwide demand for quality Ellis County cotton. Monroe Dunaway Anderson, who had arrived in Houston in 1907, used his cotton-merchandizing fortune to create a foundation that would build a medical center in Texas in the 1940s, a center that in the 1970s Red Duke would join and upon which would leave his own indelible mark.[6]

The railroad hub at Ennis had other important implications for Red Duke's story. It attracted railroad men like Red's maternal grandfather, a round-faced Irishman with jovial eyes and the unlikely name Ivo Donegan. Ivo was "Papa" to Red. Cotton and the railroads brought not only jobs for their own industries but also demand for housing and modern household appliances, which in turn increased the demand for fuels like natural gas and propane. Red's father was a first-rate salesman

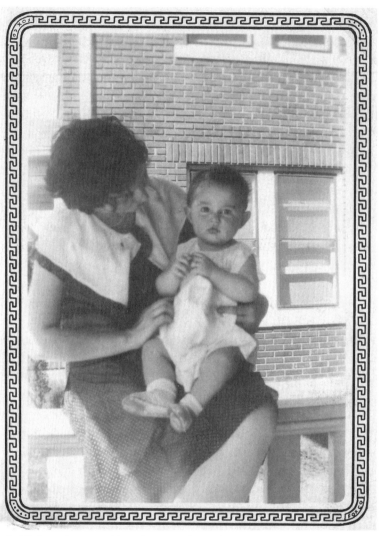

Red Duke in the arms of his adoring mother, Helen Ennis, Texas, 1929.

for the Lone Star Gas Company. Whether you needed a new stove for your house or a trainload of propane for your factory, the smooth, fast-talking Henry Duke could take care of you. So Henry Duke, the Lone Star Gas salesman, and Helen Donegan, daughter of a train conductor, would meet, marry, and find a life together in Ennis.

Growing up in that small town, Red Duke had little trouble finding his way into the local newspaper. It was hungry for stories, and no local happening—or much gossip, for that matter—escaped it. Helen carefully saved clippings chronicling events in her son's early life. "James Henry Duke Celebrates His Fourth Birthday" reads one 1932 headline. "Mrs. Henry Duke entertained on Wednesday afternoon celebrating the fourth birthday of her little son James Henry Jr. A number of games and contests were planned for the entertainment of the little folks. . . . The large birthday cake topped with white confection held four pink candles. Delicious refreshments consisting of cake and Dixie cups were served to twelve little guests."[7]

Red, who at four was already interested in baseball, is featured in another clip from the local paper extolling him as a "rising star" on the local peewee baseball team. His coach followed with a note now yellow with age, dated June 26, 1932:

Master James Duke:

You are one of our rising Baseball Stars. In recognition of this fact, I am attaching hereto a Knot-Hole Gang ticket which will entitle you to attend all the Baseball games played in the S. P. Park during the year 1932. I understand that there will be a moving picture at the Lyric Theatre soon, and this ticket will also pass you into the show.

T. F. Sullivan

Another *Ennis Daily News* mention reveals an unexpected side of Red, one he never mentioned in later years. Buried in his box of memorabilia is a clipping with "6-17-1932" penciled across the top above the headline "Ennis Dancers Appear on Dallas Circuit Tonight." The article reports that "a number of pupils of the McCleary sisters' studio went to Dallas this morning where they will appear in a program of 'Moonlit dances' which will be staged at the Texas Theatre tonight at 6 p.m."[8] Listed in the traveling dance group is James Henry Duke Jr., in the fifth number on the program, entitled "Pink Elephants." No other record of this big-city performance can be found, and any photos of the event are long lost.[9]

In another three decades, the theater in which Red Duke performed would make headlines breathlessly monitored by the entire nation. That was the theater into which President John F. Kennedy's assassin, Lee

Harvey Oswald, dashed after shooting Dallas police officer J. D. Tippet. There Oswald was apprehended and placed in custody, while Red Duke, now a surgical resident at Parkland Hospital, operated across town to save the life of Texas governor John Connally.

Not all of Red Duke's early childhood experiences were quite so pleasant as pink elephants and birthday cakes. During the same summer that he debuted his dancing talents in Dallas, Red had a serious misadventure with a lightning bug. He had been chasing it through the grass one twilight, and somehow something went amiss, and the bug flittered down into his middle ear. He had to be taken to Dallas for treatment, and his suffering was severe.

Then at seven he was stricken with pneumonia. Looking back on the experience three-quarters of a century later, he saw it like a historian. He confided:

> If you ask somebody . . . today about the crisis of pneumonia, they do not know what you are talking about, but before antibiotics were invented, pneumococcal pneumonia had its so-called "crisis," and what that meant is, somewhere between one week and ten days, if your immune system did not kick in, you died. In those days they used digitalis leaf, and that stuff grows around here. It grows everywhere in this part of the world. Some three hundred or four hundred years ago, this lady in north England found out if you ground that stuff up and gave it to people with what they call "dropsy," which was really congestive heart failure, they got better.
>
> Well, this old Dr. Clark was giving me elixir of digitalis to get my heart ready for the crisis. That is not based on any kind of double-blind, randomized trial, but he didn't have much to work with. The great thing about digitalis leaf in comparison to the pure stuff that we use now is that if you get too much of it, you see yellow and start vomiting. You cannot kill anybody with it because they cannot keep it down. Mother recognized that she was making me vomit by giving me this stuff, so she started throwing the stuff out to fool [Dr. Clark].[10]

One redeeming feature of pneumonia was an entirely different remedy—
it was a recipe made from "rock candy, honey, lemon, and bourbon," Red
told me. "I learned to love the taste of bourbon during that episode."

The town's newspaper chronicled Red's sad state almost daily for
several weeks with brief notices:

> James Duke, little son of Mr. and Mrs. J. H. Duke is detained at
> home on West Baylor Street from school with pneumonia.

> James Duke, son of Mrs. and Mrs. J. H. Duke, who has been
> sick the past week with pneumonia has developed German
> measles.

> James Henry Duke, son of Mrs. and Mrs. J. H. Duke is quite sick
> with influenza.[11]

Updates by the *Ennis Daily News* generated handfuls of get-well cards
and notes from church, classmates, teachers, family friends, and relatives. Helen, clearly pleased by the attention to her sick child, saved
them.

In time Red recovered, but not without consequence. "I know," he
told me, "[that] after that I developed diplopia, where I was seeing double. I must have had measles encephalitis, because the sixth nerve over
here does not work right. So I have what is called strabismus, which is
cross-eyed. Back then they started putting glasses on me and I started
using stuff to try to strengthen that. [We now know] it does not work
but in those days, they had the big old stereoscopes to try to strengthen
those muscles. They fix them now but they did not know how to do it
then."[12]

As a result of this condition, known to occur in about 4 percent
of the population, Red's brain had to compensate for the double image
throughout his life.[13] He would see two images, but his brain would reg-
ister them as one. His famous wire-rimmed glasses that became part
of his trademark look over the years trace their early history in part to
Ennis and a case of the measles.

Red was a good student. That fact was not always reflected in his
grades, but he loved school nevertheless. Even in the late years of his life

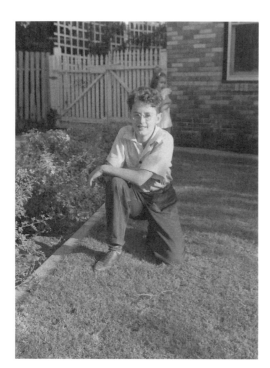

Red Duke, age nine, checking the family garden.

he could recall the names of his early teachers; he remembered these ladies (they were all ladies) in some detail and with considerable fondness. "I liked school," he told me, "and I liked my teachers. I was interested in learning and always respected classroom authority. My dad was an authority figure you didn't tangle with, so I never wanted to get on the wrong side of my teachers, [either]."[14] And he was usually in good graces. When he was out of school ill for a month when he was eight, his teacher, Mrs. Norton, who was temporarily without a car, wrote him a note: "Glad you are better," it said. "If I had some wings I would just fly over there to see you" (1935).

The year 1937 was a hard one for Red as he recovered from serious illness, suffered from vision problems, and lost weight and strength in the aftermath of the painful lightning bug attack on his eardrum. By spring things were looking up, although he had big adjustments to make, as a baby sister, Helen Patricia, came into his life. Patricia, as she would be called, was born in Dallas on March 5, 1937. Henry was making a business trip to Memphis that week; Red stayed in Ennis with the housekeeper, Lavinia.

James Henry Sr.'s neat and precise handwriting on Peabody Hotel stationery provides a glimpse into family relations at the time.

[March 11, 1937]
Dearest James,
You will never know how proud I was to get your letter today. Have been thinking of you every hour of the day and just wondering if you are being a real big boy doing what you know daddy would want you to do.
I hope you will get to see that little sister this week. I sure would like to see her about now. Went out this noon to see if I could find something she would like or rather something you would like to give her. Didn't find anything, but will get something before I leave.
I know that we all will be so happy when we get mother and little sister home. You sure are going to have to be on your toes now for that sister will be expecting you to do things for her. Sure hope your cough is better if not be sure and take that cough syrup. Tell Lavinia when they send or take our car to Dallas to take the keys to mother for I don't want the car just turned over to anyone. Will see you Saturday morning and then will have lots to tell you.
Your daddy,
J. H. Duke.

The letter suggests an easygoing nature and a sensitivity that were unfortunately not much in evidence while Henry Duke's children were growing up. His temper was explosive. Nevertheless, the letter indicates that Henry's intentions, at least, were good, and that he hoped to foster a good relationship between his children. And they had one, though it was accompanied by some teasing. There was a line that Red liked to shock adults with, and he would deliver it with great solemnity and much faked pain:

"My parents thought I might die when I was eight, so they had a replacement child. Can you believe it?"

He would pause for all the reaction he could get and then follow up with a wide grin. "And she's the pretty one. I just love her to death."[15]

Henry's promotion in May 1937 to district manager for Lone Star Gas in Hillsboro was not an opportunity to pass up in those hard economic times. Located between Dallas and Waco, Hillsboro was a larger town in which to raise a family and had more and better opportunities for an enterprising salesman. Henry was a natural-born salesman, according to Red. He was proud of that talent of his father's. Gas appliances, natural gas, propane—the word was that Henry could sell you anything. The wheeling, dealing Henry Duke was so good at sales, recalled his son years later, that he was making more in bonus pay than the president of the company was making in salary. When the company brass became aware of this state of affairs, they quickly changed the bonus formula so that the president could recover his dignity.[16]

Henry was not just a member of Ennis's Tabernacle Baptist Church; he was a fixture in it. The Baptist church ruled in the Duke household, and Red followed staunchly in his father's footsteps. He acknowledged years later that his father was a much more enthusiastic Baptist than his mother. Going to church and being involved in church were absolutes in Henry Duke's domain. "It was the center of all we did, and . . . my dad felt my success in life would be measured by my involvement and service to the church, preferably service as a Baptist preacher."[17]

As the Dukes prepared to move from Ennis to Hillsboro, the church congregation hosted a farewell buffet dinner duly reported in the town paper.

> Honoring J. H. Duke, superintendent of the Young People's Department of the Tabernacle Baptist Sunday School, who is leaving for Hillsboro to make his home, the department entertained with a beautifully appointed buffet supper Friday evening. . . .
>
> Miss Gertrude Howard, a teacher in the Young People's Department, presented Mr. Duke with a handsome magazine stand.
>
> . . . She paid a high tribute of praise to the splendid work done by Mr. Duke. . . .
>
> "How . . . Mr. Duke and family will be missed by the entire church as Mr. Duke is one of our fine, faithful deacons, chairman of the finance committee, superintendent of the Young People's Department of the Sunday School, but our loss is Hillsboro's gain and we would be greatly disappointed if we did

not feel that Mr. and Mrs. Duke would find similar places in the Baptist Church there."[18]

And indeed they did.

The magazine stand would make its way to Hillsboro with the family of four and would be filled with issues of *Life Magazine*, *National Geographic*, *Boys' Life*, reprints of Norman Vincent Peal's *Guideposts* sermons, and Henry's favorite: *Reader's Digest*.

CHAPTER 2
Family Ties

Six years before the Dukes moved there, Hillsboro had made national headlines. It was on the night of April 30, 1932. Ted Rogers and a young man known as Johnny robbed the combination jewelry store and residence of John N. Bucher. The Bucher home on County Road 4281 was just blocks north of the courthouse, and what happened next would be the talk of the town for years. While his wife stood helplessly by, Bucher was forced to open the safe. As he reached into it for his gun, which was hidden far to the back, he was fatally shot. His wife screamed in horror. The bandits fled into the dark of night with little to show for their murderous deed.

Outside behind the wheel of the getaway car was none other than Clyde Barrow.[1] Bonnie and Clyde were a national sensation during Red Duke's childhood, and the story of Clyde Barrow in Hillsboro captivated Red as he turned eight and moved with his family to this larger version of Ennis. Here tales of railroads and cotton fields had to compete with the lore of Bonnie and Clyde prowling the back roads of the Black Prairie. Although they died in a righteous hail of lawmen's bullets in Arcadia, Louisiana, on the morning of May 23, 1934, the allure and mystique of this outlaw pair from Dallas made them the talk of Red's playgrounds for years to come.

Hillsboro was surveyed as the county seat of Hill County in September 1853. It was named not for any picturesque geographical features, but for a physician from Tennessee whom Sam Houston, then president of the Republic of Texas, had appointed as an Indian agent in 1837. George Washington Hill later served the Republic as secretary of state and then as senator in the fourth Legislature, from 1851 to 1852.[2]

Hillsboro was a dangerous place in the early days as Texas settlers pushed west to the Brazos River. A general spirit of lawlessness prevailed. But after 1881, when the railroads arrived, Hillsboro became a boomtown of sorts, as Ennis had been under the same stimulus. It saw the rapid growth of churches, schools, cotton gins, mills, and stores, and it even acquired the distinction of its own opera house.

During the 1920s the town had a population of seven thousand. It benefited greatly from the establishment in 1923 of Hillsboro Junior College as part of the public school system. One of the first municipal junior colleges in Texas, it drew many educators to the area, and these redounded to the benefit of all public school students, including Red Duke, who would graduate from Hillsboro High School in 1946.

In the mid-1930s, as the Dukes prepared to relocate, Hillsboro had six manufacturers supplementing the county's dominant agriculture business, as well as businesses supporting printing and ice manufacturing. By the time Red graduated from high school, the town had thirteen new manufacturers, including new dairy processors and monument and mattress makers. It was still growing during Red's high school years, but like all the towns in the region, it saw a population decline in the 1960s as new synthetic fabrics caused a rapid drop in cotton markets worldwide.

Central to all things Hillsboro was the Hill County Courthouse.

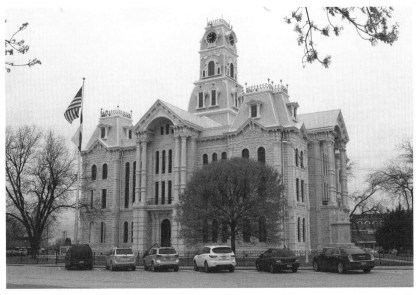

Hill County Courthouse in Hillsboro, Texas. After a New Year's fire in 1993, it was rebuilt as it stands today.

To this day the courthouse rises magnificently in the center of town. Approach Hillsboro from any direction on Texas highways and you will see from a distance that great building, the pride of Hill County. Over the years the town had replaced smaller courthouse buildings with the fourth courthouse, erected in 1890 of rusticated limestone. With three stories topped by a seventy-foot clock tower, it was one of the grandest courthouses in Texas: a Recorded Texas Historic Landmark as well as a State Archaeological Landmark.[3] The impressive edifice, along with Hillsboro's First Baptist Church just a couple of blocks away, was a central feature of Red Duke's youth,

On New Year's Day 1993, the courthouse was nearly destroyed by fire, and a statewide effort was launched to restore it. All 254 counties in Texas contributed funds, and famous sons like Willie Nelson and Red Duke pitched in as well. Benefit concerts by Willie Nelson in 1993 and 1999, with Red in attendance, helped raise money for the restoration. On May 10, 1999, George W. Bush, then governor of Texas, dedicated the immaculately restored building to a cheering crowd that filled the town's square.[4]

In the 1940s, long before the fourth courthouse burned, Red Duke

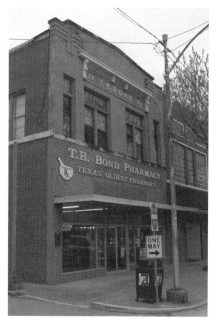

Bond Pharmacy, Hillsboro, Texas. Texas' oldest pharmacy.

was in high school. Listed on the team roster at 155 pounds, he played guard and wore number 71 for his high school football team, the Hillsboro Eagles; earned Boy Scout merit badges; and sold magazines and newspapers for future college expenses. Across from the courthouse, in Bond's Alley, Red could be found folding his newspapers many a morning before the sun came up. It was (and is still) called Bond's Alley because one of its walls is formed by the drugstore that Dr. William M. Bond established across from the courthouse in 1881. It is the oldest continuously operating drugstore in Texas.

Over the years, Bond's Alley evolved as a landmark of its own, having served as a gathering spot for Civil War veterans in the late 1800s. In Red's time it was the site of peddlers' shows, cockfights, and fisticuffs. Later it became known for an annual arts and crafts show, until finally the show outgrew the alley and moved across the street to the courthouse square.

The soda fountain at Brown Drug, one of three drugstores in Hillsboro, was a popular spot for Red and the high school crowd. In those days Red could have ordered a real ice cream soda from a "soda jerk" who knew what one was. Not far away was the Andrews Cafe, a famous landmark that in 1958 was the scene of quite a stir when a young man from Tupelo, Mississippi, named Elvis Presley, dined there.

Just down the street from Brown Drug is the Texas Theatre, where Red saw his first color movie, *Gone with the Wind*. On the south side of Elm Street was McCrory's five-and-dime. Such discount variety stores were known then as racket stores, a name originating from the racket made by metal pots and pans carried in the old tin peddler carts from years gone by. The five-and-dime must have been full of trinkets and treasures that Red, ever conscious of his college fund, coveted.

The old Del Mar Hotel, formerly the Newcomb, was a landmark gathering place in the 1940s and 1950s; there members of Lions, Rotary, and Kiwanis clubs held their meetings and banquets. And Red knew every inch of Grimes Garage. First opened in 1907, the garage was owned by one Fred Grimes, who was the first auto mechanic in Hill County. Business was slow that first year, no doubt because there were only three automobiles in the county. But in time Fred Grimes's garage grew to become an institution—it was famous for its signs placed along roads all over the country and in Europe and Asia as well. The garage

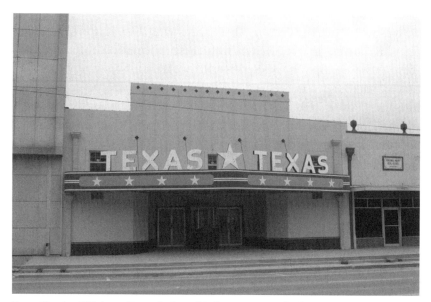

Texas Theatre, Hillsboro, Texas. Red saw his first movie in color here—Gone with the Wind.

attracted even more attention when Will Rogers said the only two things he knew about Texas were the Alamo and Grimes Garage in Hillsboro.[5]

But Hillsboro was not just an isolated prairie town with a few pleasant local haunts, a famous courthouse, and a more famous auto garage. It was a center of moderate commerce. Between 1913 and 1948, it was connected to Dallas, Waco, and towns between by the South Texas Electric Railroad, also known as the interurban.[6] And it was a place visited by the likes of John Wayne, Roy Rogers and Dale Evans, Hank Williams, and Mae West, all of whom came through Hillsboro, always drawing large crowds. On June 23, 1948, Hillsboro residents crowded a converted cow pasture on the outskirts of town, known as Bowman Field, to see a helicopter land with Lyndon B. Johnson aboard. Johnson, then a US congressman, was making a successful bid for the Senate.

And Hillsboro was further connected to the greater world by its magnificent city library. Located just down the street from the courthouse, it is still one of the most beautiful buildings in Hillsboro. Red Duke traipsed to that library many a time over the years, thumbed through its card catalog, roamed through its fragrant stacks, sat at its big oak tables, and did research for his schoolwork.

Hillsboro provided an environment that helped produce a reliable stream of people who would make contributions to the arts and sciences, to business, and to the body politic. Red Duke was one of them. So was Bob Bullock, the future thirty-eighth lieutenant governor of Texas, born and raised over at 504 Craig Street. His father was an engineer and water superintendent for the City of Hillsboro. Another Hillsboro native, Crawford Martin, who served as town mayor in 1948, would become Texas governor John Connally's secretary of state and later be elected Texas attorney general in 1966.

Texas state senator John Whitmire grew up in Hillsboro, too. His father could be found at the courthouse where he served as county clerk. Whitmire's sister Patti would marry a medical filmmaker and television producer named Mark Carlton, who guided Red Duke's television success in the 1980s. Patti Carlton recalls attending services each Sunday morning at Hillsboro's First Baptist Church and seeing the Duke family, including Red, in attendance. "His dad was an usher, and on most Sundays he could be found at the church entrance handing out the church service program. I recall Red as having a red crew cut in those days."[7]

Hillsboro's First Baptist Church was organized in 1874. Its original building was replaced in 1905 by a fine brick Greek Revival building, which is one of the city's most impressive architectural structures. During Red's high school years, his parents became founding members of a new church—Central Baptist on Old Bynum Road. "I don't know exactly what happened," Red said, perhaps somewhat disingenuously, "but there was a serious disagreement between the preacher and certain members of that flock, so my dad helped start a new church called Central Baptist Church. And Mother had not been real active until that one."[8]

One afternoon, sitting in class just weeks before his high school graduation in May of 1946, Red was assigned to summarize his life on a single page. It is easy to envision a restless Red Duke going through the motions on a lazy spring day. This was his last summer before starting college in the fall, and he was probably preoccupied with thoughts of girls, fishing, and hunting rabbits with his friends.

His single-page, penciled life history is written in uneven boyhood cursive and seems to have been hastily ripped from his spiral notebook. It is blotchy with scratch-outs and entirely unlike his precise writing in years to come. He took an easy, uninspired, bare-bones approach, beginning, predictably enough, with "I was born." Just the same, the paper is competent. It is clear, well-organized, straightforward, and free of ornamentation, and to that extent it provides a good preview of the man Red would become. And it clearly indicates what struck him at that moment as the identifying highlights of his life:

> I was born on November 16, 1928 in Ennis Texas. At the age of 6, I started [at] the public school in Ennis. Our family moved to Hillsboro in 1938. I started in the third grade at Franklin

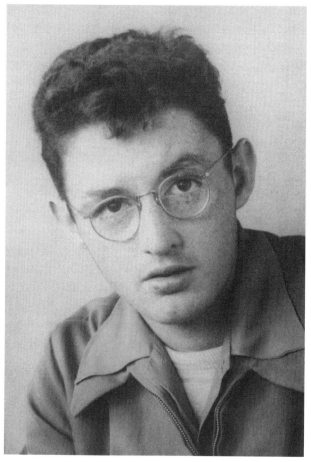

Red Duke as a high school senior headed for Texas A&M University, 1946.

School where I completed my grammar school education.
I then started Junior High School. In Junior High I learned
to play a tenor sax and became a member of the HHS band
and with two or three years experience I was admitted to the
college orchestra. About this time I came out for football for
the first time. My brief football career lasted 3 years. I lettered
all 3 years. I played basketball one year but did not continue
because of sinus trouble. I have been a member of the Boy
Scouts since the age of 12 and have become a life scout. My
last year in high school has been most enjoyable. I have always
wanted to attend A&M. I guess it's just the spirit of the Aggies
that appeals to me. It's the best.[9]

Red's musical background as a saxophone player is something few outside the family know about. Yet there is much more to be discovered
about Red Duke to better understand the literal-minded high school
student who would become an inspired trauma surgeon in the years
ahead. To appreciate the transition, it is useful to know more about
Red's parents and extended family.

James Henry Duke Sr. was a much more complicated man than
we have indicated to this point. He was born March 9, 1899, in Coleman County, Texas, the child of Welcome Smith Duke (1859–1947)
and Lelia Zelonia Cherry (1880–1953).[10] Red never knew his grandfather Welcome Duke, from Calhoun County, Alabama, because within a
year Lelia and little Henry left Welcome and returned home to live with
Lelia's parents, James Henry Cherry (1850–1930), from Linn County,
Missouri, and Nancy A. Cherry (1861–1927), a Native American of
Cherokee heritage. Mother and son would live in a small farmhouse
along with Lelia's six brothers and three sisters. While no story has
been found to explain why Lelia and her infant son left Welcome Duke,
it is known that he gave her little more than a child and the Duke name.
For Lelia and young Henry, the Cherry household would provide a tem-
porary safe haven on the family farm in Coleman.

One photo exists of the entire Cherry clan. They are sitting in stiff
chairs blandly staring at the camera with all the high seriousness of
a big family scrimping along on a small Texas farm during lean years.

"Grandpa Cherry," as Red referred to him, is front and center, somewhat awkwardly holding little Henry, who had just celebrated his first birthday. The clan seems to try to smile, but smiles didn't come easy on the dry, dusty Texas prairie of the early 1900s.

Ask an aging Red Duke to talk about Grandpa Cherry, and he would tell you the cherished family story (rumor, actually) that in his younger days James Henry Cherry had done business and perhaps even run with members of the James gang.[11] There is no evidence that Red's grandfather Cherry actually had these enviable ties to Jesse James, whose résumé included leading the James-Younger gang, robbing banks and trains, and murder, but it was a much better story than the one about Clyde Barrow in Hillsboro, and true or not, Red loved to tell it, much to the displeasure of his mother. "Brother would tell the story over and over," Patricia recalled, "just to irritate our mother as she cooked in the kitchen, trying repeatedly to get him to stop."[12]

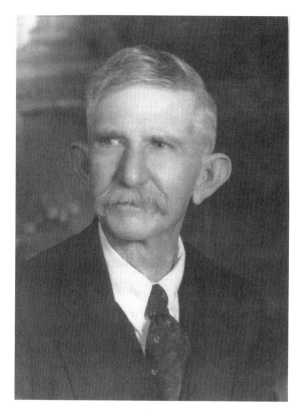

Welcome Smith Duke (1809–1947), Red's maternal grandfather who he never knew.

Hard times defined Red's father's early life. Big families were the rule, and to feed them, farmers like James Cherry scratched a living out of the ground however they could. Few, if any, in the family would finish high school in those years, including Henry.

Henry and his mother did not stay with her parents for long. By the age of six, Henry had a stepfather; his mother remarried just after Christmas in 1906, in Bell County, south of Fort Worth. Henry's new stepfather, John Henry Simmons (1876–1957), was another hard-scrabble farmer who would eke a living anyway he could to provide for his family. Lelia would have five more children with John Simmons, living on their farm between the neighboring towns of Coleman and Santa Anna, Texas.

Henry Duke was the odd man out in a household of Simmons children. He rarely told stories about his childhood, but when he did, what stood out about them and impressed Red deeply was John Simmons's vicious treatment of his stepson. According to family lore, Henry had not just been treated harshly; he had been whipped, even beaten with a chain.[13] It was a childhood he could only want to put behind him, and at the age of sixteen, he left the Simmons homestead for good. His only recourse was to religion. He turned to the Bible for comfort and hoped for a better life. He found one when he made his way to Ennis, where he met and married a beauty of Irish heritage named Helen Marion Donegan.

Helen, Red's mother, was born in Ennis on August 8, 1901. Ennis offered two major lines of work in the 1920s—cotton and the railroad, and the support services that followed them. Helen's father, Ivo Donegan (1875–1964), was born in Burns–White Bluff, Tennessee, and was a railroad man to the bone. He worked for the Texas Central Railway, later bought by the Southern Pacific. Ennis seemed a perfect place for Ivo to raise a family. On his twenty-fifth birthday, he married Rebecca Deborah Wood (1882–1967), Red's maternal grandmother, known as "Nanny." They married at the turn of the century, and a year later Helen arrived. A second daughter, Frances Elizabeth, known by Red as "Aunt Tootsie," was followed by daughter Vina and son Madison Boyd, "Uncle Boyd" to Red. Given Henry's dysfunctional childhood, the maternal side of Red's family would be his primary clan.

Grandpa Cherry of James Gang fame had died in 1930, when Red

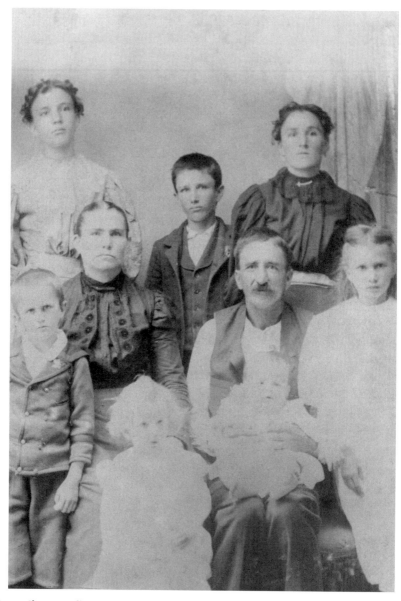

James Cherry, Red's maternal great-grandfather, holding Red's father, Henry. Given Welcome Duke (Henry's father) had abandoned his wife and young son, James Cherry provided a safe haven for Henry and his mother, Lelia Zelonia Cherry (Red's maternal grandmother known as "Nanny," in the upper right). Red's great-grandmother Nancy Cherry is to the right of James. Red loved the story, true or not, that James Cherry was once associated with Jesse James. Photo taken in Coleman, Texas, 1900.

was just two. His daughter, Red's paternal grandmother, Lelia Zelonia Cherry (1880–1953), lived in Santa Anna, Texas. Contact with her was infrequent for Red, but among his things was one letter from her, which arrived on May 21, 1946, just days before his high school graduation:

> *Dear Grandson.*
>> *I am so proud you have finished school. . . . You are real smart— am wishing you a productive future. I didn't know what to get you so will send you $100 and wish I could send more.*
> *Will close with love.*
>> *Nany.*

Nany (Henry's mother) would die seven years later, the year Red married. On the maternal side of Red's family (the Donegans), Aunt Tootsie would marry Claude Self, and their daughter, Red's cousin Claire Ruth, would be a favorite of his. Aunt Vina would marry Johnny Dubois and produce three cousins, Dick, Janie, and Helen Frances. Vina was

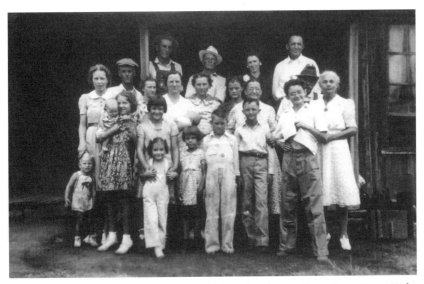

Red's Simmons clan (father's side of the family) on their farm in Santa Anna, Texas. Red is holding papers in the front row. His father, Henry, is top right. Behind Red is Henry's stepfather, John Simmons. To the left of John Simmons (far right) is Red's grandmother, Lelia Zelonia, often referred to as "Nany Cherry" by Red.

beside herself in her efforts to make her children as well-mannered and upstanding as Helen and Henry's, but Dick was a troubled young man. Vina went so far as to send him and Janie to live in Hillsboro with Helen and Henry periodically, but Dick did not improve. Letters from Henry to Red during his college years at Texas A&M and later in the army chronicled Dick's downward spiral. He dropped out of school, Henry reported, and then didn't try to get a job: "He is alright one day and the next one, he will be so hateful and indifferent" (April 6, 1952). Finally, "He and several other boys broke into Fannin school and stole a bunch of things. . . . Now they have him on probation for six months" (May 22, 1952). Dick was quickly falling from grace in the family, and no one seemed able to help him.

A photo taken on a bright, sunny day in 1946 captures the full cast of characters, with Red's "Papa" (Ivo) and Nanny, their children, and all the cousins. The prosperous clan is dressed in their Sunday best and has a soundly middle-class, professional air. The photo provides a sharp contrast with Henry's few early family photos with Grandpa Cherry and stepfather John Simmons—both of whom conjured the rural dust bowl, a world away from the Donegans. But Papa Ivo, with his round, bespectacled face and his bulldog grimace, looked exactly the part of the experienced, take-charge train conductor he was. As a conductor, Ivo did a lot more than just collect tickets. He oversaw a host of operational issues: he ensured that the train was on schedule, that the paperwork was in order, and that cars and cargo were picked up and dropped off properly. And he had to see to a miscellany of other daily business, including customer service and safety. It was a job that required organization, precision, and attention to detail—all qualities that Red's mother had and that in time Red would have, too.

And as a railroad man, Ivo was set in his ways and his opinions. It was well accepted in the family that he had perfected the art of skepticism when it came to new technologies. When John F. Kennedy proclaimed that the nation would put a man on the moon by the end of the decade and that John Glenn would orbit the earth in February of 1962, Red would listen to Ivo rant that this was not possible, that it was all a hoax, a fabrication, and a conspiracy. Ivo would go to his grave in 1966 believing that the space program was a lie perpetrated by the government.[14]

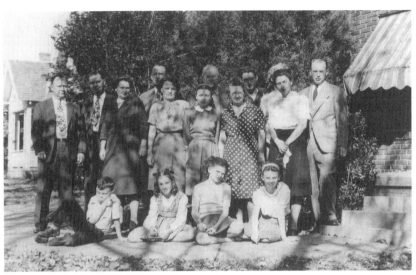

Red's Donegan clan circa 1950, composed of his mother's side of the family. Adults standing up, left to right: Claude Self, Johnny Dubois, Aunt Vina Dubois, Henry Duke (Red's father), Aunt Frances Elizabeth Self (Aunt "Tootsie"), Claire Ruth Self (Tootsie's daughter), Grandfather Ivo Donegan (known as "Pappa"), Grandmother Rebecca Donegan (known as "Nanny"), Red, Helen (Red's mother with eyes closed), Uncle Madison Donegan (known as "Uncle Boyd"), whose wife, Betty, is hidden to his right. Children sitting on the front row, left to right: Dick Dubois, Patricia (Red's sister), Janie Dubois, and Helen Frances DuBois.

He would leave behind a railroad man's sense of responsibility and devotion to service, as well as the organizational skills and penchant for timelines and detail that Red would take note of and benefit from. And he instilled in Red a sense of adventure, a longing to see places far beyond Ennis and Hillsboro.

A penciled Christmas request from a seven-year-old Red to Santa on December 23, 1935, provides evidence of another interest Ivo stirred in Red's developing imagination:

Dear Santa Claus—
I want things for my electric train. Please bring me an oil car, a lumber car and a caboose. Please Santa Claus bring me a box of

signals setting up—not hooking on the tracks—also two switches
and additional tracks. Thank you and Santa Claus—I am going to be
a good boy.
Yours truly,

James Henry Duke, Jr.
605 W. Baylor
Ennis, Texas

Nanny Donegan outlived Ivo by three years. She lived with Red and Betty and their children during the final year of her life, and when she died in 1967, her pride in her grandson, the doctor who cared for her in his home until the end, was boundless.

CHAPTER 3
Lessons in Life

Every good deed a man does is to please his father.
—MAX PERKINS

Red Duke loved his devout Baptist father, the wheeling and dealing, community-minded, consummate salesman Henry. And on the surface, Henry was an ideal family man. Both his children were well-adjusted, outgoing achievers. They never drifted or lacked purpose or direction or wandered into trouble. To whatever extent he was responsible for the way his children turned out, Henry was a successful father.

Yet he was far from a perfect one. Henry had baggage of his own from a childhood in which he never seemed to have a real home, one that he felt was rightfully his and in which he felt fully welcome. He lived with his mother's family in his early years and later with his stepfather, John Simmons. By all accounts, Simmons never seemed to accept Henry Duke into his household, and consequently Henry never had a real father figure. He felt not just unappreciated but resented, and he was no stranger to the rod. When he became a father himself, he was bent on being a good one, but he was without a role model. And his childhood had left him with a vein of anger, even rage, that made him hard to live with when the front door was closed. This deacon of the Baptist church and pillar of his community could be tyrannical at home—intolerant, demanding, and loud. Patricia suffered acutely from his storms, whether they were directed at her or not, and when Red left for college, Henry's fuse grew shorter and his explosions grew louder. "Brother never knew this," she told me, "but life was hell afterwards." It had not been particularly pleasant before, either—including for Red, because Henry was "very hard on my brother."[1]

Helen was the counterbalance who stabilized the household. She must have suffered deeply from her husband's anger, but she tolerated it dutifully, minimized it as much as she could at home, and protected

Henry's upright image in the town. Red rarely talked about this side of his father's character. He accepted the bad with the good and focused resolutely on the good. But the suppressed memories hovered in out-of-the-way corners of his mind; once, deep into the night, he confessed to Betty, fists clinched, "Sometimes I wanted to kill him." But for the most part Red dealt with Henry's demons palliatively, even humorously. One way he mitigated them was by manipulating family devotional time each morning.

On one occasion, when Red was home from seminary for the weekend, Patricia, a cheerleader, had been at school helping decorate the gym for a Halloween dance. On the way home, another car struck hers as she pulled away from a stop sign. Terrified at the prospect of facing her father, she nevertheless had to call home. "And he came down there," she said.

> He was screaming like a madman and Brother came with him. Of course, I was a basket case. Just put me away. I thought I would never drive again.
>
> Well, we go home—not one word was said in the car, and I was sitting between Brother and Daddy, scared to death. We get home. Lunch is ready. We all sit down, and Daddy says, "We have to say the blessing." And Brother stood up and said, "Let us pray." And he prayed a prayer that would not end—a prayer that was the prayer of all ages—a prayer you would not believe. Brother and I laughed about it for years, because he shut my dad up with a prayer. I escaped his wrath and Mother, of course, was in shock. Brother thought that was the funniest thing. He was a true big brother watching out for me that day.[2]

At least Henry's explosive temper taught Red lessons in deflecting bad behavior.

Henry taught his son other lessons, too, and fortunately they came from a better place. One of them was the value of work: "My dad certainly knew how to raise a boy, keep him working and tired all the time," Red asserted, and with approval.[3] For Henry there were no doubt practical benefits to keeping his son busy, but he also believed in the moral benefits of working long hours and developing discipline—preferably more discipline than he possessed himself. Looking back, Red would often comment on how he had worked all his life, because that is just what you do. "I have grown up with kind of a work drive—I think probably to please my dad."

Red's work drive covered working for free, working for pocket money, and even working for pansies. "In Ennis as a child there was a fellow's flower shop about three hundred yards from our house, the Dunlap Flower Shop. I used to work there potting plants. . . . I was just a kid, a little kid, but they paid me in pansies, which I adored. I thought that was the best thing going."[4] What he actually wanted with the pansies was to give his mother a bouquet. He chose the flowers that went in it himself.

Patricia also remembers that her brother was always working: "To be truthful, he was pushed by my dad, but maybe that's good. Look where he ended up. He would pick cotton, dig postholes, ditches, anything to make a little extra money. I would go out to pick him up with Daddy, and there they were, dragging those big white cotton bags."[5]

Today the Hillsboro Outlet Mall occupies the open fields where Red once picked cotton. Looking back on his cotton-picking career, he acknowledged that "for sure I was not a very good cotton picker. Others around me were like spiders with hands going everywhere in constant motion filling their bags."[6] But what he lacked in speed and dexterity he must have made up in determination, because he kept picking cotton.

Much more lucrative for the enterprising redhead were newspapers and magazines. Patricia remembers that "Daddy would take all the boys at four o'clock in the morning to the alley behind the drug store, and they'd bag up their papers to take them all over town." Red was a young entrepreneur, according to a local newspaper article in 1942:

> It takes a heap of book-keeping, says 14-year-old James Duke of Hillsboro, to keep up with his man-sized job of handling the *Dallas Morning News* agency for his town. James is just the boy who can do it, however, and that's why he was chosen to succeed the previous agent who retired.
>
> James, son of Mr. and Mrs. J. H. Duke of Hillsboro where his dad is Lone Star district manager, is clearing about $60 a month, part of which goes in the bank toward his college education. . . .

James has four boys working for him. Gets up before day-light every morning to check his papers out as they come in on an early interurban. Sundays there are 480 papers to throw and through the week 368 every morning. He also sells Texas almanacs and has already taken orders for better than 100 copies. . . .

Working, James still finds time to make the honor roll at Hillsboro high school where he is a sophomore. He is also a Star Scout and active as a leader in the Hillsboro Council. He plans to attend A. & M. and study engineering.[7]

The scouting that the Hillsboro paper took note of was a profoundly influential part of Red Duke's youth. The Boy Scouts contributed greatly to his proficiency as an outdoorsman and consequently to his being as well balanced as he was. Scouting provided him with practical skills that served him well in all his many undertakings, and he was still devoted to it even in the last years of his life. Red Duke loved the Boy Scouts.

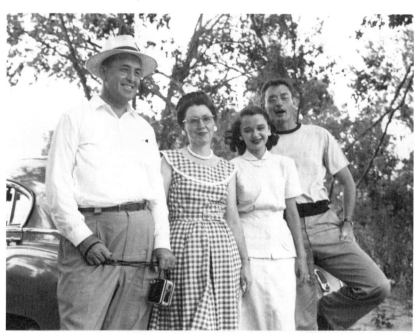

Henry Duke and family: Helen, Patricia, and Red. Hillsboro, 1948.

Trustworthy, Loyal, Helpful, Friendly, Courteous, Kind, Obedient, Cheerful, Thrifty, Brave, Clean, and Reverent. These twelve words outline the qualities every good Boy Scout is expected to exemplify.[8] Duke tried to live the values of scouting throughout his life. He was never hesitant to remind any audience, however rarified or sophisticated, how much scouting had meant to him. To the twelve Boy Scout virtues he added one additional trait that he preached daily to anybody who would listen: common sense.

Joining the Boy Scouts when he was twelve brought Red new father figures and adult mentors, as well as organized adventures that stressed developing skills and pursuing competitive goals to move up in the scouting ranks. In time he would advance from tenderfoot to second class, first class, star, life, and the prize that most scouts aspire to but few achieve—Eagle Scout. In 1946, his senior year in high school, Red became an Eagle Scout.

Four decades later, in 1986, he would be recognized by the national Boy Scouts of America as a Distinguished Eagle Scout, an honor he considered to be among his highest accolades in life. The distinction is available only to Eagle Scouts with twenty-five years or more of outstanding community service and has been won by such men as Neil Armstrong, Steven Spielberg, Ross Perot, Donald Rumsfeld, William Westmoreland, and Robert Gates.[9]

As he advanced steadily through scouting during his high school years, Red honed his leadership as well as his outdoors skills. He added to his collection of merit badges, which are earned through focused work and demonstrated accomplishment. Merit badges for camping and fishing came easy. Those for first aid, lifesaving, and conservation added new prospects from which to survey possibilities for his life ahead.

Red had just joined the Scouts when the Japanese bombed Pearl Harbor.

I can remember exactly where I was. . . . I was playing football on a Sunday afternoon on Louie Marshall's lot. He had a big-sized lot. This is when everybody got in gear. It was a remarkable and memorable moment. . . . We had three scout troops, and we had a competition to see who could get the most scrap metal together. They were collecting scrap metal for the war

effort and bins were placed down on the courthouse square. If
that metal was not welded down, you'd be damn sure somebody was going to get it. The whole country was gung-ho. We
started those Victory Gardens and I certainly remember pulling weeds out of the garden. Lord, I thought that the Johnson
grassroots went to China; it was hard to get rid of them.[10]

Through scouting Red developed and honed survival skills. He camped
in wilderness settings, learning to live off the land, to pitch tents even
in the middle of the night, and to start a fire with flint and bark tinder.
Additionally, he made new friends at district events held beyond the con-
fines of Hillsboro. And with great determination he pursued advances
in rank by earning merit badges (twenty-one were and are still required
for the Eagle rank).

The acquisition of certain merit badges left lifelong memories. Pursuit of the poultry-keeping badge in particular did that, thanks to an
angry chicken with a superior sense of timing. "One of my many daily
tasks in the morning was to go out and feed, water, gather the eggs,
and rake the henhouse," Red recounted. Evidently he grew bored with
the mindlessness of the chore—"You know, raking the henhouse is not
an intellectual challenge"—and he lost his temper with a hen who had
remained on the roost and wouldn't come down. "And I started hollering at her. Apparently she was standing in some feces and kicked it up
with her wing while I was hollering. I'll never forget the taste of that
stuff going down my throat. So I quit raking and went to spitting."[11]

Scouting to Red was partly about piling up merit badges and trying to achieve Eagle rank and the Order of the Arrow, but it was also
about the reality behind the badges. It was about learning the trait of
resourcefulness and about contributing to the community in ways that
would be meaningful to his father. Red always wanted to leave things
a little better than the he found them—whether a campsite, a community, or, in time, a patient. Scouting gave him a powerful sense of confidence and accomplishment; it fueled his trajectory forward and was
a source of pride to his family. Red was not just any son, but an Eagle
Scout on his way to great things.

As a good scout, Red knew the history and loved the story of a lost
American in London in the early 1900s. He was rescued by a cheerful

boy who refused compensation, saying that he was a Boy Scout and could not accept payment for a Good Turn. A Good Turn, the boy explained, is a volunteered kind act or deed that you don't have to be asked to do and you don't seek attention for.

The American was a grateful Chicago publisher named William Boyce. Boyce was intrigued; he pursued more information, and on February 8, 1910, he formed the Boy Scouts of America.[12] It was Boyce's gift for the Good Turn he had been given that foggy morning in London.

In 1912 *Boys' Life* magazine was first introduced as the official publication of the Boy Scouts of America. Red filled Henry's magazine rack with eagerly awaited, well-worn issues. A story in the issue dated July 15, 1916, which was more than a dozen years older than Red himself, still made the rounds in Hillsboro. The town's first troop had started just a year earlier and had made the big time with this national mention in the magazine. It continued to be a source of hilarity: "There is a scout in Hillsboro, Texas, who will get a merit badge in angling if he keeps on. One June day he went swimming with other scouts and caught a fish in his bathing suit. He did not intend to, and he was very much surprised, not to say scared. If the swim to the bank had been timed by officials he would have a world's record to his credit."[13]

Boy's Life not only refined Red's practical skills and leadership abilities; it also opened his eyes to a topic that would become an enduring passion—namely, wildlife conservation. Every issue of the magazine included standing headlines with examples of conservation practices that other boys were involved in across the nation, and Red took note: "Meadville, Pennsylvania scouts planted 5,000 white pine seedlings on a tract of land owned by the Meadville Water Works Department"; "The Utica, New York Fish and Game Protective Association conducted a prize essay contest and also a bird house contest for the local scouts"; "Altoona [Pennsylvania] scouts have planted thousands of young trees on the watershed supporting birds and wildlife at Kittanning Point, where the city obtains its water supply."[14]

Issue after issue of the magazine provided examples of such conservation efforts, not just in concept but in action—constructive conservation projects that appealed to the values of young Red Duke, who would, in 1986, be named president of the Boone and Crockett Club, the famed national organization founded a century earlier by Theodore Roosevelt.

Conservation was a major focus of Red's adult life. He invested time, money, and energy in his commitment to it.

Teddy Roosevelt, a personal hero of Red's, not only championed conservation throughout his life, but was also an ardent booster of the Boy Scouts movement and served as troop committeeman of Troop 39 in Oyster Bay, New York, and first council commissioner of Cassau County Council.[15] Roosevelt was the first and only man designated by the Boy Scouts as Chief Scout Citizen.

The notion of a Good Turn took hold of Red Duke's imagination and never let it go. Red came to believe that the Good Turn really represents a philosophy of living, one in which service defines you. Red's life would be full of Good Turns; opportunities to perform them seemed to come his way unsought daily. And of course when he became a surgeon, helping other people became his way of life.

The stories of two of his Good Turns found their way to his parents' ears at home in Hillsboro in the form of unexpected letters. The first is dated February 23, 1952. It was written to Henry and Helen by C. A. Shockley, a stranger who lived in Oklahoma City and had met Red on a train. Red and the recipient of the Good Turn were both bound for College Station, "I, to see a son stationed there," wrote Shockley, "and Jim to get his commission. I became very ill on the train and Jim was kind enough to help me. In fact I don't know what I would have done without his help, just wish there were a million of young Jim Dukes. You know most young folks do not care anything about elderly folks, but that cannot be said about your son, he is one of the best."

A few months later Helen received the second letter singing Red's praises. While he was stationed in Germany, he had gone on leave to Salzburg to call on an elderly cousin of his mother's, Martha Clark, who lived in California but was visiting abroad. On May 15, the surprised old lady expressed her pleasure in a letter to Helen. Addressing her as "Mrs. Duke," she writes:

> Last Sunday, Mother's Day, will be a delightful and charm-
> ing memory to me always. Your son Jim and John Clark were
> responsible for giving me this utterly spontaneous and happy
> day through their unexpected visit, totally unpremeditated
> and real. I have a son in New Zealand and I know I would be

proud of him if he went so out of his way to be kind to an older person whom he might never see again. You have a jewel of a boy in Jim. I think he will go far and bring great happiness to those who cross his path. . . . I felt both boys were fine and superior young Americans and it made me feel proud of my country, proud of them, and proud of *you* for rearing such a son.

Red Duke had grown up in a small Texas town, in a strongly religious household that promoted a Herculean work ethic, and under what was for him the powerful influence of the Boy Scouts. He seems to have been genetically endowed with good nature and generosity of spirit and more than his rightful share of energy. He was set early on a path toward a lifetime of Good Turns and service. This is not to say he lacked streaks of waggishness that got him into trouble a respectable number of times. And there would be world enough for that in the years ahead. But first, after graduating from high school, he needed to stretch his wings beyond Hillsboro and do something few in his extended family of Dukes, Cherrys, Simmonses, or Donegans had done before him—go to college.[16]

CHAPTER 4
A College Man

On May 28, 1946, the *Hillsboro Evening Mirror* led the news with a banner headline about the national coal strike that was the talk of the country. The headline below was local and on a happier subject: "111 Receive College, High School Diplomas Monday." Red was one of eighty-four seniors graduating from Hillsboro High that night in Doughty Hall. (The other twenty-seven graduates were from the junior college that shared the campus.) The class valedictorian, Bob Beavers, incorporated the big issue of the day, the coal strike, into his discourse, which was titled "Selfishness—Pitfall of Mankind."[1]

For Red, as for most graduating seniors, the moment was rife with both joy and trepidation. He had finished the first obstacle course on his way to adulthood, and his life was about to change radically. More and tougher obstacles lay ahead, but his sense of accomplishment was immense. He could feel his parents' pride as they sat among their friends and neighbors to celebrate the moment. Patricia was also there; just two months earlier the family had celebrated her ninth birthday. Most of Red's extended family, and his own parents, had never gone beyond high school, making this evening even more important, because for Red it was a springboard into college. Most of his relatives were poor Texas farmers with many mouths to feed, little money to feed them with, and not much education. High school, much less college, had with few exceptions simply not been an option for most of the family.[2]

Red—Eagle Scout, football letterman, band member, hardworking teenaged newspaper and magazine entrepreneur—was different; he was on his way to places other family members had never aspired to reach. World War II had ended just more than a year earlier, and things were looking up everywhere. Gas was no longer rationed, which was particularly good because Texas A&M was some 120 miles from Hillsboro. A small amount of money could make the difference between being able to get home when he wanted to and being stuck on campus.

As he sat in Doughty Hall that night, Red was looking forward to a summer of hard labor. He would dig ditches and postholes for Lone Star Gas. But college was his ticket out of a whole lifetime of manual labor. Spending time doing things that would tend to dismantle his body was not appealing. That was especially the case after a tackle earlier in the year during a football game had left him unconscious on the field with a concussion. He thought he would prefer to work with his head. It was, fortunately, still intact, although when he regained consciousness after the football mishap, "They just sat me up, cleared my head, and put me right back in the game. Concussions didn't get much attention in those days."[3]

He wanted an engineering degree, and A&M was the place to go for one. "I am a frustrated engineer," he would claim years later. "All through A&M I was struggling with that problem, and I took a lot of science courses and I took a lot of business courses too. Growing up I was building airplanes all the time. If I found an old chicken crate, I'd build something."[4] What kind of engineer he wanted to be isn't clear, but perhaps he was practicing for civil engineering when he tried to concoct dynamite. "Drugstores were interesting in those days," he said. "You could buy paregoric, which is just opium off the shelf, for diarrhea, and you could buy sulfuric acid, nitric acid, and glycerin. I kept trying to make dynamite. I could make all the black powder stuff you wanted, but I never was successful—I tried but I never could. I don't know what Dr. Nobel did to make it work, but I didn't. It is a good thing, too."[5]

Looking back, he also recalled that one of his father's employees at Lone Star Gas had a son who was planning to go to medical school. "Somehow I got medical school in my craw, and I don't know why, but I really could not be a doctor. I had to be a preacher, and I did not want to be a preacher. It's what my dad wanted."[6] Henry the strict Baptist deacon made it clear that dreams about engineering and medicine were folly; the greatest good Red could achieve in the service of others was as a preacher. If James Henry Duke Sr. could be a Baptist deacon, James Henry Duke Jr. should be a Baptist preacher. But for the moment, A&M and a bachelor's degree stood between Red and that unsatisfactory prospect.

Texas A&M was the state's first public institution of higher education. It was established as a direct consequence of the 1866 Morrill Act.[7]

That post–Civil War legislation provided for the donation of public land to the states to fund higher education, whose "leading object shall be, without excluding other scientific and classical studies, and including military tactics, to teach such branches of learning as are related to agriculture and mechanic arts." In 1876 the Agricultural and Mechanical College of Texas, or Texas A&M, opened its doors, and instruction began that same year. Admission was limited to white males, and military participation was required of all students. A decade after Red's graduation in 1950, changes were made allowing the admission of women and minorities. And the once mandatory participation in the corps of cadets became voluntary.[8]

With the war over, Texas A&M saw an unprecedented enrollment in September 1946. Virtually two-thirds of the new students were World War II veterans. "Enrollment was limited," A&M president Gibb Gilchrist advised incoming students, "so that all Texas veterans who were entering college for the first time, all former students of the college, and all June graduates of Texas high schools would have a place at A&M."[9] Even so, the college had to turn the Bryan Army Air Field into an annex. It was a busy, exhilarating time.

Red chronicled his college years through letters home, and a great

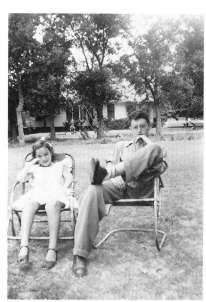

Red with his sister, Patricia, home in Hillsboro during college, 1947.

many of these were saved by their recipients and came back to him later in life, after the deaths of his parents. They provide insights into and periodic snapshots of his college years that otherwise would be lost. The letters are for the most part hurried. They are not introspective—they tend to the narrative rather than the reflective and have more to say about what their author was doing (and eating) than what he was thinking. To that extent they can be frustrating. But they are often funny, and the bedrock of humor is insight. Red thought more deeply than he admitted. He simply didn't talk about thinking. His letters often were committed to campus stationery that featured rival football games with slogans and cartoonish art showing Baylor Bears being stomped by the Aggies, or poor Bevo, the mascot of the Longhorns (a longhorn steer), running for his life to escape the all-powerful Corps of Cadets.

The Texas Longhorns' first mascot, in 1914, was a dog named Pig Bellmont in honor of L. Theo Bellmont, the university's first athletics director, and Gus "Pig" Dittmar, who played center on the football team. In 1916, Pig the Dog was replaced by the 1,200-pound Bevo, who was so obstinate when he was first dragged onto the field that students described him in the school newspaper as "the most recalcitrant freshman ever bulldozed into higher education."[10]

Red loved all the stories about spirit, tradition, and college rivalries. He did not suspect as he entered Texas A&M that one day he would be a Longhorn—a professor at the University of Texas in its medical school at Houston. Always a dog lover, Red was more than content and not even slightly conflicted during his college days to cheer on his team, admiring A&M's less massive mascot, a collie named Reveille, as the dog raced along the sidelines of the football field.

A letter home dated October 9, 1946, reports on Red's highest priority during his first semester—food. "This morning, Spider [Red's longtime friend from Hillsboro, Allan Eubank] got hold of a bunch of cans of milk and drank seven, I believe. He was almost as full as I was the Saturday I was at home. Oh yea, that reminds me, we can get plenty of food usually if we start meal-hounding at the right time. I got hot cakes, syrup, grape nuts, toast & jelly, eggs and bacon and coffee. This was an unusually good one."

The demands of exam schedules and coursework also compelled his attention:

Boy—it seems like the courses get harder by the week; freshmen are beginning to drop out fast. We've lost two of them this
week. Burks almost left this morning but has decided to stay
on. . . . Boy I wish we didn't have to go anywhere but home on
week-ends, just to see the family, eat, and be just a little lazy. I
really enjoy shooting the breeze with homefolks. [But] I think I
learned some damn good lessons since I've been down here—
this place is pretty good place for a fellow to be—I think. I'm
telling you the food gets worse each time we eat, and less of
it too. That home cooken is really good, it used to be swell but
now—Ohhhhhh Brother!! Better get to studying for a trig quiz.
Love, Red (October 31, 1946)

During the early part of the semester, Red's letters had been about football games, new friends, and the wonderful times he was having with
his newfound freedom. Then, as the weeks wore on, he began to talk
instead about how little time he had to study and how difficult academic
life was proving to be. He knew that at some point his grades would find
their way home, so he took steps to cut the news off at the pass. He may

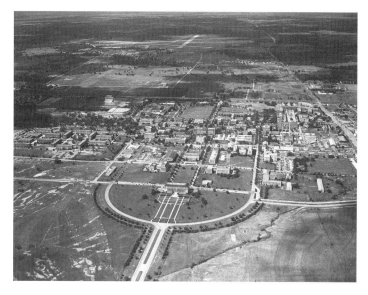

*Texas A&M University in College Station, Texas, as it looked in the 1940s when Red was
a student. Courtesy of Cushing Memorial Library and Archives, Texas A&M University.*

have made the honor roll in high school a time or two, but college was a new day.

> Oh yea—when you get my grades—I may have a D in Trig— that's a mistake—I made a 76 in the course which entitles me to a C–. Don't get in no uproar over that. I was doing alright until he pulled that stinking quiz on us and gave us a problem we had never had. . . . We have been getting bout five hours sleep lately. . . . Better get to studying—so long. Love, Red (November 14, 1946)

As the Christmas holidays and first-semester grades grew alarmingly close, Red's letters home took up a complaint that in hindsight is laughably ironic, given that the day was coming when he would be a professor himself and the inspiration for similar letters home from his students. "I'm telling you," he grumbled, "the professors are getting more chicken by the day, all they want to do is try and make us get bad grades" (December 4, 1946).

The grade report for the first half of Red's first semester away from home was dated November 7 and directed to Henry and Helen in Hillsboro. That would be one weekend Red was not anxious to drop by for mom's home cooking. Two As (orientation courses), five Cs, and a D in trigonometry.[11] President Gilchrist sent a message home to the parents of every freshman, saying that he hoped their student had "done acceptable work. If he has not, he should be given every encouragement to put forth a greater effort so that by the end of the semester his grades will be acceptable."[12] Red's father no doubt took this generic advice to heart. He would have had more than a few words ready for his son during the Thanksgiving holidays.

The irony of Red's less-than-stellar grades as a freshman and sophomore in college was that in years to come he would be first in his seminary class and second in his medical school class. He was academically gifted and highly capable. At the same time, he was a social animal who preferred campus life to the classroom. Whether he changed his preferences as time went on is doubtful. What changed was his performance.

During his sophomore year Red decided to resurrect his football career. He made the university's B team (junior varsity), and one result was even more demands on his time. His letters home, which had once filled four pages, now filled one or two:

[September 5, 1947]
    Dear Folks,
    I'm kinda tired—won't be much of a letter. It's a great life—rough and hard but great if you want it. It's been awfully hot—we work out (106 yesterday) from 9:15 a.m. to 11:30 a.m. and from 4:00 pm to 6:30 pm. I'm still kinda sore but am coming out of it slowly—we scrimmage nearly every day and are supposed to have a game with the varsity on Sat. Lord only knows when I'll be home—we eat good.
    —Red

Although football made new demands on Red's time, it satisfied his love of comradery and his joy in new friends, competition, and school

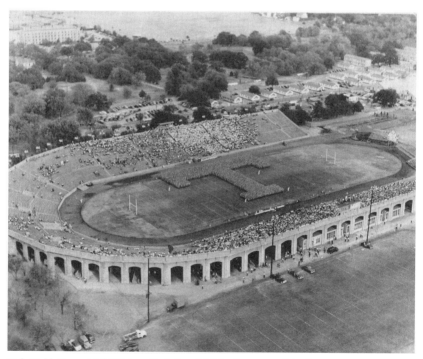

Kyle Field, Texas A&M University in late 1940s. Courtesy of Cushing Memorial Library and Archives, Texas A&M University.

spirit. For the junior team, there were no fancy team buses and escorts to games. Red's description of a twenty-four-hour road trip by car to a game in Baton Rouge captures the spirit of the day and shows why his grades suffered. Leaving College Station just before noon on a Saturday, the teammates had more than 750 round-trip miles to cover, along with a nighttime football game. The uncomfortable return overnight was followed by Monday morning workouts and class.

The trip was not improved by the condition of Louisiana highways at the time. "That state," Red wrote, "ain't no good. Dust, fog, smoke, bad roads—they never seen a bulldozer over there. We got in Baton Rouge just in time for the game—we couldn't find a place to stay so we took turns driving back—came back by Beaumont, Houston. Somewhere this side of Beaumont we ran into a forest fire—we had to drive with the door open to watch the black line—got back about noon Sunday. That is about it. A full 24 hours. I've got to get some studying in" (October 14, 1947).

But he loved every minute of a trip like this—an adventure filled with tight deadlines, unexpected detours, and fly-by-the-seat-of-your-pants crises.

In addition to football, there were the constant demands of the corps of cadets. This meant uniform pressing, boot polishing, dorm inspections, and more. But Red also loved this military side to his college life, especially as he advanced into his junior and senior years. The tradition and spirit that ruled football and the cadet corps were exactly why he had chosen A&M in the first place.

Sometimes rules got in the way and had to be nudged aside. A report sent by the Office of the Commandant to the assistant dean of men reflects an instance of such nudging. Red had just written home that he had acquired a puppy. He had added, without specifics, that "she's quite a mess." Days later the report appeared:

SUBJECT: Dog in Dorm 2.
    TO: Assistant Dean of Men.

    1. The dog mentioned in the Battalion is the one the janitors have been complaining about in Dorm 2.

2. Red Duke states that the dog has disappeared, and if it should return he will not take it in the dorm again.

[Signed]
Marion P. Bowden, Lt. Col., Inf. Tactical Officer[13]

Red kept Lt. Col. Bowden busy. A second report, typed and filed the same day, reads:

SUBJECT: Student behavior: James H. Duke, N. R. Patterson
TO: Assistant Dean of Men.

1. Cadets Duke and Patterson said that they had been studying late, and the course was on laws for preventing fires in public buildings. They learned that a fire hose should be 100 feet long and they didn't believe the one in Dorm 2 was that long. They went down to measure it when the Patrolman came in. After he took their names and the story they measured the hose and put it back in the rack. The hose was 75 feet long. Also they stated they were not up to any pranks.
2. In view of the above statements and the fact that they were not up to any pranks or damaging of college property no action is necessary.
3. I recommend that the college pick up this fire hose.[14]

By his second year, Red's favorite road trips always included a stop halfway home, in Waco. He and his buddies didn't miss a Baylor varsity football game if they could help it. Red looked forward both to the games and to meeting students unlike any to be found on the A&M campus—specifically, girls. At football games in Waco, Red was obviously watching more than the game on the field. He reports as much to his parents (in precariously dated language): "There was a good crowd and lots of felines too—they looked good cept for those long skirts and black hose" (October 28, 1946).

In another letter home dated just after Christmas in his sophomore year, it is clear that girls were still on his mind, particularly one named

Nancy, whose mother and aunt brought her to a dance in College Station in a 1946 Lincoln convertible. "Lovely thing (the car)," he joked before sending his mother into a real tizzy: "Sit down mother—no, maybe you better lay down and let dad sit down. She had a pair of the prettiest lips you ever saw. I said it—and I'm glad. . . . I know you think she's just the first gal I seen in a long time—but for some reason I had the best time at that dance. Hope she enjoyed it much as I—doubt it though. I'll tell you all about it later on sometime" (December 25, 1947).

Red was clearly smitten with Nancy, but in a future letter he's still talking about the Lincoln convertible—about Nancy, not so much.

Not every letter was upbeat. When one of his roommates dropped out of school, Red's spirits took a dive. The dorm was just not the same. "Kind of sullen around here," he wrote. "Dreary day. They are working ol' Red hard. Better get back to my studies" (November 19, 1947).

He made the choice between engineering and a business degree in late winter of his sophomore year. Engineering had little appeal:

> I'm telling you the farther I get into this engineering stuff—the more I say to myself I'm not cut out to be one—I really believe it too. I believe I could graduate an engineer from A&M (don't know how long it would take me) but I'd have to work like the devil all the way just to get by. . . . But you all know me well enough that I'm not made to be content starting now and spending the rest of my life . . . doing one thing. No lie I work all the time I can find—after taps some, all weekend, study periods, off periods—but I just can't seem to do any good. (February 18, 1947)

It was a turning point, but more a turning away from something than toward something. Red was still uncertain about his future direction. He explored industrial education and then settled back on the path to a business administration degree. He continued to be content with mediocre grades, especially during his early years at A&M, because he intuitively understood that his time at college offered an opportunity to enjoy life in a carefree way that would not present itself again. Everyone who knew him described him as friendly and outgoing. Already his charisma could attract a whole room.

As Red turned away from an engineering degree and confessed in letters home that his football career was not going well, he increasingly turned his attention to the regimented activities of the corps of cadets. His letters home during his junior and senior years increasingly talk about his polished boots and the satisfaction of dorm inspections that went well, a visiting colonel he had found an opportunity to chat with, and the value of a disciplined approach to life. His grades improved noticeably.[15]

Red had chosen A&M to revel in the school's spirit, and he could hardly do that better than as a yell leader. The Aggie yell leaders are a select group of students elected by the student body. There are only five of them: three seniors and two juniors. Together they use a variety of hand signals called "pass-backs" to direct and intensify the crowds. Election to yell leader is one of the most coveted honors on campus.

According to university lore, Aggie yell leaders represent a tradition dating back to 1907. The Aggies were being soundly defeated at a football game, and many of the girls at Texas Woman's University in Denton (near Dallas) were threatening to leave the game early. The upperclassmen, who had imperial (and enforceable) authority over freshmen, ordered the freshmen to think fast and not let the women drift away. They had to make them want to stay, however badly the game was going. Several freshman, so the story goes, located some white janitorial coveralls. Hurriedly pulling them on as uniforms of a sort, they rushed out onto the field with improvised yells spiced with jokes. The performance was hugely successful—the girls must have stayed—and thus was born the Aggie yell tradition.[16]

However, the Aggie yell was so popular, especially with the girls, that it was snatched away from the innovative freshmen who had dreamed it up. The upperclassmen appropriated for themselves the privilege of leading yells, and they are still in possession of it.

Red waited for his opportunity as a junior to audition. He must have been thrilled when he learned in a letter from the dean that he had been elected, and he must have felt vindicated in his decision to give up the football team. He would have more attention as a yell leader than he would have had as a mediocre football player, and none of the bruises. And yell leaders are among the few students who qualify for a varsity letter without playing a sport.

Now the gregarious Red Duke could be seen at all the Aggie-sponsored sporting events and university-wide special events as a representative of the values and spirit of the university at large. The high school senior who had written about going to A&M because he liked the spirit there was now the voice and presence of that spirit. He gleefully accepted his new responsibilities and tried his best to stay out of trouble, in keeping with this new distinction.

Some days, however, he fell short.

Baylor University students had a chant, "Beat the Aggies, beat the Aggies, beat them black and blue." They would do it over and over again. Well, I was sitting up in the third floor of the administration building, and why I can remember all this I do not know, but I was in Dr. Delaplane's South American Economics class, and I guess I was doing that just trying to figure out what I might do for a living, and I wrote this poem using that line, "Beat the Aggies, beat them black and blue." It was inflammatory, but it was not vulgar. The trouble is, I did not have any money. There was a guy here, a famous fellow who was a consummate Aggie, the class of '32, and his name was [Judson] Loupot, who ran this little shop selling used books and used uniforms. All Aggies knew him. I went up there and told him I needed a little bit of money to get this printed, and he spent twelve dollars to get about a thousand of those things printed on gold paper and in green ink so it would look like somebody from Baylor wrote it.

We had one kid. He was a sophomore from San Antonio. He had an airplane. We were going to fly at night and deliver them all over campus (inciting our Aggie campus on a grand scale against Baylor), and he decided not to do that, which was wise. But he had a car, and he was one of the few people that had a car, so he distributed them that way with some other guys and the campus cops caught them. I was not going to let them take the heat, so the next morning I remember very clearly cleaning up and getting the best uniform I could get on, and I turned myself in to administration as the guilty party. I

ATHLETIC DEPARTMENT

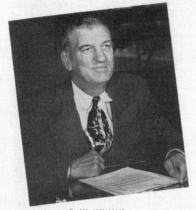

D. W. WILLIAMS
Chairman, Athletic Council

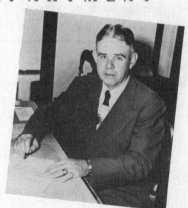

BARLOW "BONES" IRVIN
Athletic Director

YELL LEADERS

Front row: Glenn Kothmann, head senior yell leader.
Middle row: James "Red" Duke, senior yell leader, and William "Tex" Thornton, veteran yell leader.
Back row: Don Joseph, junior yell leader, and Bill Richey, junior yell leader.

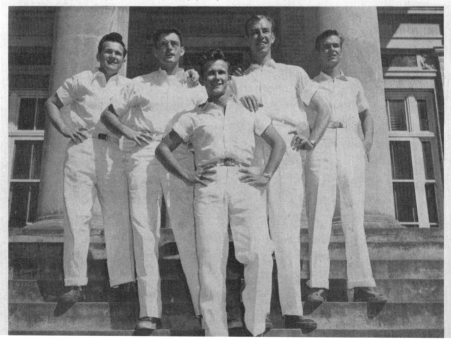

Red Duke (second from left) as senior Yell Leader at Texas A&M University, 1950.
Courtesy of Cushing Memorial Library and Archives, Texas A&M University.

have never seen anybody so mad at me in my life—thought for sure I was going to be expelled on that one.[17]

Unfortunately Red did not reveal the ditty that so inflamed the powers at A&M. He said only that it was "inflammatory" but "not obscene." Perhaps Red's idea of an obscenity differed from the administration's. Perhaps it was something political; the war wasn't long over, and the Japanese were great droppers of propaganda from planes. These flyers were not dropped from a plane, but they looked as if they had been. What unimaginably awful political ditty could a student as popular as Red Duke have penned and distributed on campus that would have nearly gotten him expelled? Littering was not a hanging offense in 1948.

Whatever this literary transgression was, it was clearly pretty bad. News of it—or some version of the news—evidently leaked home. To stem whatever tide of wrath was likely to be forthcoming, Red had his girlfriend at the time, Jane Dennis, write his mother. "He wanted me to tell you," Jane wrote cautiously, "that 'the trouble' he was in last weekend—it's alright. He ought to know by next weekend what the outcome is. He said he would write about it but didn't want to worry Mr. Duke" (October 30, 1948).

Red escaped expulsion. For what, we don't know. It is consoling that there were a thousand flyers. However, few were distributed before the police showed up; someday one will surely surface.

Although even in his eighties Red Duke still wouldn't quote his "Beat the Aggies" ditty, he did lay claim to the Baylor "bearnapping." And while many people have claimed to be the perpetrators of that deed, Red's story is more convincing than most. He said that he came up with the idea to steal the mascot and talked some freshmen into the ploy. To his surprise they pulled it off, creating quite a stir on both campuses.

Red, as the story goes, decided someone needed to return the bear to Waco. Once again, as instigator, he recruited some freshmen for the deed. It would be a challenge, given that the bear was in the news and was probably not in a cheerful frame of mind. Not having a car, Red's accomplices borrowed a fellow student's station wagon, leaving out a few details about the intended passenger. The bear was returned to Waco in the dark of night, and the borrowed vehicle found its way back to College Station well-chewed and pooed.

Once again Red turned himself in as the mastermind of the misdeed and was threatened by the school's administration with permanent expulsion. Fortunately, his case was reviewed by his peers—student government officers who in the end no-billed him. His college life was saved. One can only wonder which was harder—getting the bear safely back to Waco or keeping his mischief and near expulsion from school out of earshot of his father, who no doubt would have roared louder than the mascot.[18]

Red Duke's senior year would be a good one, with his passion for trouble tamed for the most part. He was the senior yell leader, and he took the increased responsibility of the position to heart, even starting a notable school tradition of his own. He was the first senior yell leader to read "The Last Corps Trip" at bonfire.[19] The reading of that poem at bonfire became a Texas A&M tradition for the next five decades and was a source of pride for Red throughout his life. At his funeral service, the school's senior yell leader made his own appearance in full whites to honor Red with a reading.

A major change for Red as a junior and senior was his sharpening focus on the military side of his schooling. Going into his final year of undergraduate studies, he had a busy summer schedule, not in Hillsboro, but at Camp Hood, where he participated in the Army ROTC summer training camp in Killeen, about one hundred miles from College Station, due north of Austin.

Here more than eight hundred Army ROTC cadets from across the country came together between June 18 and July 30 for intensified training. Competition was keen among the colleges participating and the cadets seeking individual recognition and honors.[20]

Camp Hood, renamed Fort Hood in 1950, was officially opened on September 18, 1942, and has been used for armored training ever since. The army base was named in honor of Gen. John Bell Hood of Confederacy fame. During World War II, as many as one hundred thousand soldiers trained for war at Camp Hood. During the latter part of the war, some four thousand German prisoners were interned there.[21]

If you wanted to learn how to drive a tank and fire heavy artillery, Camp Hood was the place to be, and Red Duke did and was. This was no

Football Begins...

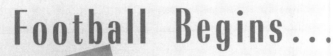

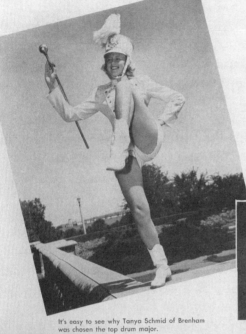

The year began in earnest. The Ags played Villanova under Kyle Field's new lights on September 17. Over 30,000 people, the largest opening game crowd in A&M's history, turned out to see the game and watch high school bands from all over the state strut their stuff.

It's easy to see why Tanya Schmid of Brenham was chosen the top drum major.

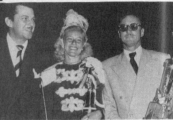

Glenn McCarthy presents Tanya with a trophy while movie star John Carroll looks on.

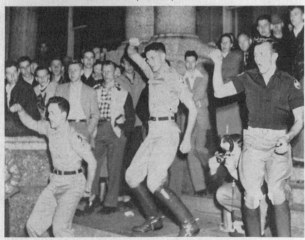

The first yell practice of the year starts things off right. Glenn, Red, and Don lead the troops before the Villanova game.

198

Red Duke, senior Yell Leader during his senior year at Texas A&M. Courtesy of Cushing Memorial Library and Archives, Texas A&M University.

classroom exercise or campus drill. Camp Hood was the big time. As a kid with a BB gun shooting at cans and other makeshift targets with his friends along the banks of the Aquilla Creek, Red had never imagined that any guns could be so big or make so much noise.

Red found army life harder than cadet life, though he minimized the difference—it was, he said, "a little on the rough side" in comparison. The noise of the guns was huge; perhaps it contributed to his increasing deafness in later life. "All these dang guns" going off was, he reported home, especially painful for the tank commander, because he had to stick his head outside the tank to "see where the round hit and make corrections. Inside the tank it's alright—doesn't bother you at all." And, "You just can't imagine the flame behind the explosion" (July 13, 1949).

Here in the 2nd Armored Division, Red Duke was learning to be a tank commander. He was learning to shoot the big guns. He had found something on a scale big enough to fit his interests. The practice and the discipline it required, and the danger and the competition, were all to his taste. If he was going to do something, the bigger and bolder, the better. Commanding a tank was right up there. (And it helped to compensate for all his failed youthful attempts to make drugstore dynamite.)

That he enjoyed this army life was one thing. The question particularly relevant to Duke, though, was whether he excelled among his peers at it. The lead headline of the A&M campus newspaper, The Battalion, on the morning of August 1, 1949, provides the answer: "Duke Is One of Seven Outstanding at Hood."[22] The article reads: "James H. 'Red' Duke, senior yell leader for 1949–1950, Friday was named the outstanding cadet for Company G, cavalry, at Camp Hood during final

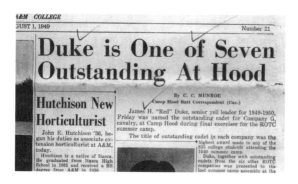

Newspaper article detailing Red's outstanding cadet distinction at Camp Hood.

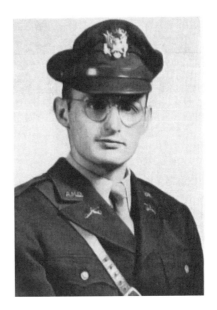

Tank commander Lt. James Duke Jr. Courtesy of Cushing Memorial Library and Archives, Texas A&M University.

exercises for the ROTC summer camp. The title of outstanding cadet in each company was the highest award made to any of the 835 college students attending the 1949 summer camp."

As both a senior yell leader and the outstanding cadet during summer drills, Red was off to a resoundingly good start in his senior year. These honors inspired him with confidence and gave him a profound sense of self-satisfaction. Letters home that final year show a self-assured young man on the move, successful in everything he attempts. The letters also reflect his pride in the military aspect of his student life. He comments that his boots are polished, inspections go well, and he "really get[s] a buzz out of those tanks" (February 16, 1949).

At the end of the school year in 1950, Red took possession of his bachelor's degree in business administration and his coveted Aggie ring.

But something else had come in the mail to Hillsboro as he was driving tanks around the armory courses of Camp Hood: a United States draft card dated June 22, 1949, and stamped "Status 1A." With college complete, it was time for Red to address his military service.

CHAPTER 5

Tank Commander

Red's success at Camp Hood fueled his desire to get into the US Army. Already his buddies from A&M were in active service. But as he awaited his own call to active duty, Red Duke did exactly the opposite of what everyone (with the exception of his father) expected him to do. He enrolled in seminary.

The school he chose was Southwestern Baptist Theological Seminary in Fort Worth. Red took this drastic step, which violated his own expressed wishes for his future, purely out of a sense of filial obligation. He did it to please his father. His parents approved of preaching in churches; they did not especially approve of driving around in large armored weapons bent on destruction. But the seminary doors had no sooner clicked shut behind him than Red began to regret his capitulation. He earnestly did not want to spend his life on the business end of a pulpit.

This had been a false start, and almost immediately he moved to correct it. He put in a request for a tour of active duty. It came very quickly, and Red withdrew from seminary, packed his bags, and returned to military life. Whether he requested active duty with Henry's knowledge or did it surreptitiously is open to question. But if Henry was ignorant that Red had volunteered, he could have seen this return to the military only as a no-fault defection from seminary.

Then, astonishingly, after going on active duty in May 1951, by June Red was already at work trying to get back into seminary, or going through the motions of trying to. In an undated letter (to which he received a reply dated June 17), he appealed to Dr. Alfred Carpenter, the director of the chaplains commission for the Southern Baptist Convention, to help him get a leave of absence in order to return to seminary and complete his degree. There followed a long exchange of letters between the army and representatives of the Baptist church to get Red discharged from active duty and returned to seminary.[1] In the end, the wheels of military bureaucracy moved slowly enough that Red would never get discharged from active duty this way and would finish his service out as a first lieutenant in the US Army Cavalry and not through the chaplains commission.

If this comedy was a result of uncharacteristic indecision on Red's part, his letters from the period could be expected to show signs of some sort of interior distress. They do not. They are entirely typical of his usual balance and good spirits. There is every evidence that he heartily enjoyed army life and the opportunities it gave him to enlarge on his experience—to meet new people, go new places, do new things.

Another explanation for the whirligig of activity is that, even if he did not know about the request for active service, Henry was so unhappy over the brevity of his son's skirmish with seminary that Red soothed him with this charade. Or Henry found out himself about the loophole and put Red on the spot. In any case, the correspondence with the military and the chaplains commission did not trouble Red—most of it was conducted by other people, and when he had to take a turn at the typewriter, he did not even correct his spelling. In short, he appears to have carried on his duties and his recreations oblivious to the background drama.

• • •

The army's officer training school for tank commanders took Red Duke outside Texas for the first time, to the rolling hills of Fort Knox, Kentucky.[2] He enrolled in the required basic officer training course to become an officer in the cavalry. He took eighteen weeks in basic soldiering skills, maneuver tactics, troop- and company-level strategy, and logistical planning. Here he would be able to put into use everything he had learned in A&M's cadets program. He would master organizational and leadership skills for getting big jobs done with whatever resources were available.

Red's delight in army life is evident in his letters home. Things began to roll even on the first day of class. "We spent the morning on administrative problems of the motor officer and the afternoon on field expedience," he wrote Patricia.

> Now just what is field expedience you ask? I'll tell you. It is the
> practice of employing the most available material and equip-
> ment at hand when some unusual incident occurs when in
> an area not occupied by any other equipment or facilities that
> would aid in solving a problem. Some examples of the situa-
> tions would be a tank stuck with no other vehicle there to pull
> him out or say for instance a jeep with a wheel shot off and no
> spare tire. All these problems have a solution. You must always
> be able to find an answer to a problem. (May 31, 1951)

For Red this was invaluable training that would have significant applica-
tions to surgery later on, for in medicine as in the military, unexpected
problems often demand innovative solutions. In another letter home,
he pointed out new lessons he was learning about leadership, or, as he
may have thought of it, being the boss: "Today we did nothing more
than clean up tanks. At least the men did. I was the assistant officer of
the day and put in charge. I can't get accustomed to the fact of having
someone do everything I tell them. You sorta have to watch what you
tell them" (April 5, 1951).

As he would always do, Red turned his downtime to good use. On
one occasion he went to the Indianapolis 500. Pecking out a letter to
Patricia (whom he addressed as "Hi Sweetheart") on the small portable
typewriter that went everywhere with him, he recorded the winning
speed, which was "500 miles in 3 hours, 57 minutes, and 38 seconds.
That's pretty fast for an airplane, much less an automobile. If nothing
else the opportunity to see those beautiful cars was a thrill." There was
another thrill, too. "For your information, Loretta Young was there to
award the winner with a trophy as well as a kiss. (I have even thought
of taking up driving now.) She had on a lovely snow white dress that
couldn't have looked better anywhere at any time. That lady has
beauty."

Not to let any free time get away from him, he planned another
excursion for the weekend: "Since I don't have anyone to visit . . . I think
I shall go down to Mammoth Cave after church Sunday and take a
tour. . . . All my life I have heard of the 'Cave.' I had no idea that I would
someday actually have the opportunity to see it." And, perhaps inspired
by his sight of the pulchritudinous Miss Young, he added, "By the way,

don't let any of the cute ones get married till I return from the great war. Remember, I am still a bachelor—pretty eligible too" (May 31, 1951).

Writing home to Henry, he described the cave in terms his father would appreciate. It was a "magnificent spectacle" that was "truly a work of God Almighty." Henry, no doubt, was pleased to hear Red in such a reverent mood. But the Baptist deacon, anxious for his son to get back to seminary, may have been less pleased with other parts of the letter. His army training school was, Red said,

> the Holy Land for regular army armored officers. You see this is the place where they develop all these ground force weapons, equipment, and tactics. This is truly a great fortress of freedom from the military viewpoint. I wish [we] could see some of the things they are working on now that are only the test stage. They have one new tank up here that will someday be our heavy tank in the 2nd Armored. It's the biggest thing I have ever seen. I have no idea how many tons the thing weighs. I used to think that the M-46 tank was large, and it is for that matter, but it doesn't even hold a candle to this new one. I know one thing for sure, it has a 120 mm gun on it.

But, knowing that his father would be less enamored than he was of the destructive power of the bigger and better tank, Red returned to a topic likelier to meet with paternal approval. "I'm going to make it a point to attend one of the Northern Baptist churches Sunday," he promised, "and see just what the real story is. That is something that I'll include in the next edition" (June 1, 1951).

Having bought a used car, Red was mobile, and he took every opportunity to see the sights on weekend leave and reported every trip in his letters home. He was always bent on sharing the pleasures of travel with his parents. And the letters seem to record an itinerary that fulfilled youthful promises he had made to himself. Sometimes they seem rather like notches cut triumphantly into a gunstock. For example, he recounted his impressions of the sights in and around Cincinnati. The Ohio River Valley was "as green as anything you have ever seen or read about. Scattered all along the road are these beautiful palatial country homes bordered by those famous white board fences." Coney Island amusement park was memorable principally for offering a glimpse of Patti Page. The Beverly Hills Country Club was elegant—"so pleasant, so refined." The Taft Museum, original home of the Taft family, impressed him with its fine paintings. An Episcopal church service met with his approval because of its prayerfulness.

He described a breakfast at a cafeteria in Ohio; he was rapturous over the small, wonderful Ohio strawberries that came with it. ("Now for a fact they have us beat in that respect.") Then, sounding almost like a caricature of an exemplary son, he writes, "After picking up my little water-marked Bible from the breakfast table I set out to find myself a church to attend that beautiful Sunday morning. After some reconnaissance, I located the toll of chimes in my ear. It was not the Northern Baptist Church that I had wanted to go to; it was a beautiful old Episcopal church" (June 13, 1951). This was the church that so recommended itself to him by the fact that worshippers knelt in prayer instead of praying from the pew.

Red continued his weekend road trips with buddies who counted

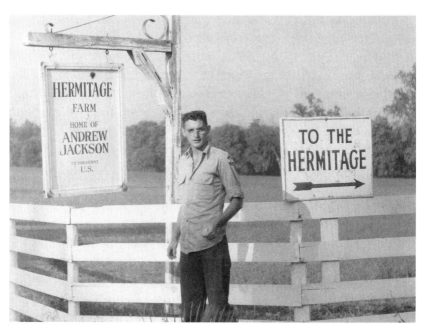

On the road with Red Duke, who spent every spare moment during army officer training in Fort Knox, Kentucky, seeing places he had only read about.

themselves lucky that he had a car. His nonstop determination to see the sights at every available opportunity continued unabated. But he found that letters home were just not doing the job. "As I can see it from here, Old Red has some real experiences ahead of him yet that would be of extreme interest to you all. What do you think of getting a motion picture camera upon which I can record for you all the many things that I see?" (August 2, 1951). In time Red bought a still camera and sent home film for the family to process to supplement his letters. But the pictures are not mentioned in Henry's letters, and he may not have been keen on paying to develop the film. Neither pictures nor film have come to light.

Meanwhile Red's weekend forays opened his eyes to more of the country. He wrote letters home describing such new discoveries as Cumberland Falls; the Natural Arch Bridge; Gatlinburg, Tennessee; and "what I consider the greatest cathedral I have ever seen, that great range of mountains—the Smokey Mountains. I cannot remember when I have been so shaken by such beauty" (August 2, 1951).

• • •

Red had been destined for Korea, where the war was raging. But in early November of 1951 he received orders deploying him to Germany. "I don't know why—I ought to look it up because I've said what I am about to say a jillion times—we were on our way to Korea[,] so I thought. I do not know what the Russians did but all of a sudden they moved the Second Armor as fast as they could to Europe. I was still in Kentucky [in training] but as soon as I finished that, I went to Europe."[3]

He awaited final orders in Camp Kilmer, New Jersey. From its opening in 1942 through the end of World War II, Camp Kilmer was a major transportation hub for US soldiers traveling to and from the European theater. During the war years, more than 1.3 million servicemen were staged at Camp Kilmer before deployment in Europe.[4] Here while he cooled his heels, Red entertained himself by taking advantage of the many rail lines that left the base for major East Coast cities. This was a far cry from the interurban electric rail connecting Hillsboro to a handful of Texas towns.

He was stunned by the fall colors. Splendid reds, yellows, oranges, they were unlike anything he had ever seen in Texas. He took a Saturday train trip to Philadelphia to watch a football game pitting the University of Pennsylvania against the University of California, where he sat on the California side of the stadium. "I saw Governor Earl Warren, his wife and three blonde headed daughters of which we have seen so much of in *Life Magazine*," he reported to the family at home (October 3, 1951). Earl Warren would resurface in Red's life twelve years later, when he chaired the famous Warren Commission on the assassination of John F. Kennedy in Dallas, an event in which Red would find himself involved as a surgeon.

As the year sped to its end, the cold northern climate asserted itself. The temperatures dropped, and Red, who never liked cold, shivered and grumbled. Army regulations would not allow furnaces on base to be lit until temperatures dropped to specified levels, and Red waited impatiently. "Thank the Lord tomorrow is the day set for the fireman to fire up the furnaces," he wrote. "I can hardly wait." Then, repenting lest he alarm his parents, he mitigated his complaint: "Let me hasten to stress the fact that I am not being mistreated or allowed to freeze for I definitely am not, nor am I unhappy or [is] my morale low. I am just a bit chilly" (October 9, 1951).

Although his surviving letters are largely silent about his responses to New York, where he sometimes went on weekends, the city must have left him agape, as it does everyone who first comes to it, at its immensity, the variety of its people, the food, shops, buildings, the traffic, the subway, the crowds. He was especially struck by the Church of St. John the Divine, which he stopped to admire for half an hour. "This is an Episcopal Cathedral," he told his parents, "which has been under construction for the past 55 years and is only two-thirds finished. When finished it will be the largest stone structure in the world" (October 9, 1951).

Another foray led him to New York Penn Station, where he met and fell into conversation with a fellow officer who, he discovered, shared his ambition to ride the subway to Yankee Stadium and watch the sixth game of the 1951 World Series. The defending champions, the New York Yankees, were pitted against the New York Giants. Red and his new friend had intended to buy tickets, but he reported home that two police officers stepped up and offered them free tickets to the game. The Yankees won, and Red always remembered the kind gesture, the Good Turn, these two officers in blue provided two unknown soldiers.

Red told the story in his letter home and sent along his reserved ticket stub for the upper deck, showing a purchase price for a Yankees World Series ball game to be all of six dollars that year. Red and his new-found army buddy watched the Yankees on their way to winning the series—their third straight title and fourteenth overall World Series victory at the time. For someone who enjoyed seeing a celebrity, as Red always did, the series was a real treat; it was the last World Series for Joe DiMaggio and the first for two unknown rookies named Willie Mays and Mickey Mantle. Of course, he had to enjoy Mays's and Mantle's celebrity later, in retrospect.

In Washington, DC, for the first time Red came to appreciate real traffic. "Now more than ever before I can understand why the people of the eastern states don't travel anything like as much as we do," he said, and tried his hand at prediction: "I can really see why the railroads will prosper in this section for a long time." In Washington he also got together with an old roommate, who introduced him to "some of the famous government girls." He may have had rather too good a time. In any case, indulging in his curious proclivity for talking about people his own age as if he were vastly older, he declared Washington unfit for young women: "I have come to one solid conclusion. . . . I shall never allow any young lady [for] whom I am responsible to go work alone in that city. . . . That is no place for a young person to go without some strict leadership" (October 20, 1951). Whatever prompted this opinion, his three daughters decades later found it highly comical.

When he was not waxing philosophical on the dangers of DC, Red made haste to "see as much as my eyes would let me which [was] of course directly dependent upon my two feet which were the media of travel." He would happily spend hours in the Smithsonian museums on the Washington Mall. The Lincoln Memorial was a favorite, too. "This is truly a beautiful tribute to the man," he wrote, "very very impressive" (October 20, 1951). During this interlude Red received word that the army would not release him from active duty to return to seminary. His reaction does not seem stricken, since seminary was Henry's ambition, not his. "I cannot feel too badly," he wrote to his father, "nor can I rejoice upon the news. . . . All in all we know that whatever the Lord does is for the best, our main concern is to seek his divine will for us and be satisfied and happy wherever he places us" (October 10, 1951). Of course, it was easier for Red to submit to the will of God in this matter, since it was identical to his own. But Henry was not a man to give up, and Red remained peculiarly—almost inexplicably—susceptible to his influence. The story was not yet over.

• • •

For a young man like Red Duke to see the sights of Washington, DC, and New York City was one thing. But to set sail in uniform for the distant shores of Europe was another—something he had probably scarcely even dreamed of growing up in Hillsboro picking cotton, selling magazines, and hoping to one day get to Texas A&M. But to experience the delights of Europe, first he had to get there, and that would prove an uncomfortable task, and a smelly one.

On November 5, 1951, Red deployed to Mainz, Germany, on the USS General M. B. Stewart, a 522-foot squire-class transport ship with 2,471 soldiers and crew on board. The accommodations for dining were decent; those for sleeping, less so. The ship's dinner menu for November 14, 1951, which Red saved, suggests better-than-adequate fare for the trip from New York to Bremerhaven via Southampton: grilled lamb chops with "piti" pois, arroz con pollo, Boston seafood chowder, mashed turnips. Dessert was strawberry shortcake.

The conditions Red's men encountered below deck were rather unpleasant.

> To the best of my knowledge the day is Wednesday, the 14th day of November. We are sailing just off the coast of England. I was given a compartment of 56 men, compartment E-3 that is. In that space of about the size of our living room at home, 56 men have been living. . . . They sleep in bunks four deep. That first morning that I went down there to get them ready for the inspection that we have every day, I became a little discouraged. Every one of the fellows was deathly seasick and up top side. If you all have never seen a person that is seasick, then you have an experience that I hope you never witness. To date I've not succumbed to the plague but it is hard sometimes. After about four days they got their sea legs back. The sailor that accompanies the Commander on inspections says that

we have the sharpest compartment on the ship. It just goes to prove that if you will just hold on, it is bound to get better. . . . The stench that a ship acquires after a few days at sea is terrible.

Perhaps thinking back wistfully to his days at A&M when he was measuring the dorm's fire hose to see if it met code, he adds a final pronouncement on the ship's condition. "I sometimes think that it would have been wise to get some pictures of the conditions that existed in the compartments during the first few days for further reference. I'd like to start another little congressional investigation myself" (November 14, 1951).

Red's letters home from Germany were prolific and filled with all the detail and description he could muster. To the relief of his family, no doubt, he resorted increasingly to his trusty portable typewriter. His handwriting had always been hurried and hard to read. Typing, he could write more and with greater pleasure to both himself and his correspondents. Now he could truly be the eyes and ears of the family,

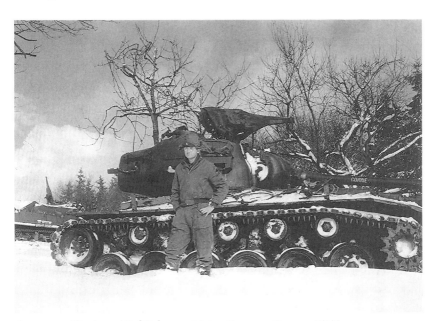

Army second lieutenant Red Duke near Mainz, Germany, January 1953.

seeing and hearing a world that his parents and sister at home might never otherwise experience. They awaited his letters eagerly. Henry even suggested at one point that the letters should be numbered to ensure that none went missing.

Red spent seven months in Germany. His working life consisted of awaiting orders, moving men and tanks around on German rails to meet the demands of practice maneuvers, and continuously performing and overseeing tank maintenance. He found the work tedious, and he suffered from homesickness at times and from some disagreeable living conditions. ("There is a terrific wind outside. They say that it is supposed to get up around 60 mph tonight. This attic room may get blown off if we aren't careful" [January 2, 1952].)

Red managed to find time during his assignment to see the towns of Mainz, Munich, Garmisch (where he took his first lesson on skis), Baumholder, Nuremberg, Berlin, and Berchtesgaden, and the Buchenwald and Belsen concentration camps. He also managed to fit in Salzburg, Austria. He described all these places in detail sufficient, he hoped, to make his parents and his sister feel a real experience of them.

Red settled into the responsibilities of a tank commander watching over his men and responding to orders. He also taught courses on tank maintenance and enjoyed it. But he especially liked being in charge. He soon had an opportunity to command in the field when a new lieutenant, supposedly in charge, seemed to be traveling more than leading.

> I have decided that the only answer is to have a lot of
> patience[,] for that young gentleman is going to hang himself.
> We have been here about two weeks and that young fellow has
> found excuses to be in Mainz for eight of those days. About six
> of those eight days your red-headed correspondent has been
> the acting company commander. . . . I think the job of the
> company commander is the greatest in the army for learning
> about people. They come crying to me with every problem in
> the world and it gives me every opportunity to exert judgment,
> common sense if I have any, and to be firm when necessary.
> It is really great. He is gone now and I hope he doesn't come
> back until we go in. I really like having my own little kingdom
> figuratively speaking of course where I can operate in the

way that I feel is most efficient and beneficial to all concerned.
(February 5, 1952)

Letters home included vivid descriptions of churches he had visited. His detailed descriptions of tank drills and the firepower of new tanks that shook and pounded his body while taking a toll on his hearing no doubt worried Helen as she read page after page of his long, typed letters. "I'm deaf as a post," he would often remind people in his later years. For those who had read the letters describing tank drills, his hearing loss later in life would come as no surprise.

His letters to his parents often express gratitude for his Texas A&M years and his cadet training there. It gave him a strong jump-start for army life in Germany. His Boy Scout experience also made a difference. He credited "a little Scout initiative" for helping him solve a sheltering problem by rigging a tarp to the tank's track; it provided a snow shelter for his men. "The new quarters are dry and warm," he reported home proudly, and included a detailed drawing of his innovation (November 14, 1951).

One cold night in February 1952 he typed a philosophical message to his cousin Jane Dubois, who was living with his parents and sister in Hillsboro at the time. Jane's brother, Dick, continued to have problems with the law, according to updates from Henry, but Jane had just finished high school and was thinking about college. Putting on his big-brother hat, Red offered his younger cousin advice gleaned from his own life experiences.

One point to Miss Dubois. I love your letters, but sit down and write me one telling me specifically just what you want to study in college, where, and for how long you are willing to study. Remember this young lady, you aren't going to get it all done in a big hurry and the more difficult it is for you, the better it will be for you as you will be a better person when your goal is achieved. And that brings up another point, set yourself a goal, a high one, maybe one that you can't quite reach, but something that you can always strive for. And above all, regardless of the circumstances, Red is with you. (February 5, 1952)

The last sentence is touching. It rings true, even though the reader is aware that Red will probably not think about his cousin again until a letter from her or one about her from his parents recalls her to mind. But when she does come back to mind, his impulse will be as generous as when he closed the letter: "Red is with you." The same generosity of spirit seems to have guided all his relationships, including the one with his father.

Henry, the frugal salesman always looking for a get-rich scheme, wrote repeatedly with ideas like one he had about bamboo fishing rods that Red might buy in Europe at bargain prices, ship home, and sell in Hillsboro at a tidy profit. Red was much less interested in financial wheeling and dealing than in buying his mother a set of china. Fortunately Henry was interested in doing that, too, and few letters during Red's seven-month stay in Germany escaped a mention of the china—how to get the money to Red, what color (cobalt blue was Red's preference), what pattern, how many teacups. An endless stream of details consumed Red as he made plans to buy a lifetime gift for his mother.[5]

The letters between father and son about the great china purchase all end with a new idea left hanging for further discussion. Time began to run out, and in the summer of 1952 Red was put on orders to return to the states. A frantic letter arrived home; project china purchase had to be executed immediately. "Now dad," Red wrote, "if you have ever done anything that I really requested, please comply with this one. Take all the money out of the savings account that you said that you had been placing there and also cash those bonds that are due now and wire the money to me. This rush is not good, but we will have to make the best of it" (June 1, 1952).

Helen's china was finally secured, and Red was on his way home. If nothing else, the china had taken Henry's mind off his black-market schemes and off getting Red back to seminary, at least for the moment. But in the spring he had written a letter entreating Red to reconsider seminary. His argument appealed to an opening of his paternal heart, to piety, and to the authority of spiritually minded men. He also offered a small bribe in the form of an extra month of travel.

It is so difficult for me to really express what is in my heart. But I want to again try to give you my idea, since you asked me to. Just to lay the cards on the table and pray the Lord that you will take this as it is meant. I don't feel that the Lord would see that your studying all about tanks—big guns and all the machinery the army has, would help you in preparing yourself to win souls for his Kingdom and if this was my opinion alone then I would be more hesitant to express it to you, but all that I have talked to that I think are men who think of spiritual things first, express a like opinion. And that is why I am so convinced that you need so much to get back in school, and into the real job that is ahead of you. And here has been my thinking along that line, that you apply for a release as suggested by Dr. Newman [of Southwestern Baptist Seminary, who had been lobbying to get Red released from the military through the chaplains commission], and if it goes through any ways soon, then you take some 30 or 40 days and do all the traveling you see fit to, before you grab a boat back for the U.S. But try to enter Seminary this fall. And if you would go on and make up your mind I think we could get this through where you could do that. Now please pray and think this over. (April 6, 1952)

Why Henry wanted Red to keep trying for a release from military service through the chaplains commission makes little sense, because he would be released very shortly anyway. Perhaps he thought this route would commit Red to seminary and the chaplaincy. Perhaps he thought it would prevent him from signing on again as a tank commander.

Henry longed for "one of those old-time bull sessions" with his son. Without naming the offense, he apologized for the rages that had shattered the peace of home for many years:

We could exchange ideas freely and I think could understand them much better than by letter. I do appreciate more than you will ever know, the kind words you said about your old Dad, but let me tell you this my boy, I look back now and see so many things that I would like to correct, or things that I would

handle different from the way I did then, or would have been
more tolerant and understanding than I was. But at the time I
thought I was making the right decision. So please forgive me
for all my blunders, and I will do my best to make up for them
in the future. (April 6, 1952)

Red's tour of duty in Germany as a second lieutenant in the US Army
ended on its own accord with a promotion to first lieutenant and without special discharge from active duty. He left Germany in June 1952
and was sent back to Fort Hood with the 4005th Replacement Company
to be discharged around July 18. His official army diploma bearing the
imprint from the office of the president of the United States documented
the completion of his service to his country—it arrived in Hillsboro a
year after his return to the states and was dated August 18, 1953. Red
would file his military records in the box of memorabilia dating from his
childhood. Now it included his stint as a tank commander.

His return from Germany in the summer of 1952 marked an important crossroad. It was the beginning of a new chapter in Red's life and
presaged a major decision. Would he make a life in the church, or would
he pursue his own path?

CHAPTER 6
Seminary Hill

When Red Duke was released from the army, he enrolled in seminary, not medical school. That is not what he wanted to do—he had already rejected seminary once. So why, at the end of that summer of 1952, did he go back? He treated the question with the loquacity typical of him when questions got too close to the core: "I came back," he said, "and the conflict still existed, so I started seminary."[1]

The reason, of course, was Henry. Henry had not-too-subtly, but also not-too-infuriatingly, promoted the ministry to Red for two decades. He was convinced that preaching was the highest calling and that the ministry more than any other profession would make Red's life meaningful. Religion had made his own youth as an emotionally abandoned stepchild bearable, and later on it had provided structure for his life. Perhaps in his eyes he owed God a debt—even saw Red as a sort of oblate, a gift to God, one that would attest to Henry's own faith and redound to his glory. Perhaps it would wash away—even vindicate—the rages he had visited on his family during the years when his children were growing up.

Putting a son into the ministry would affirm to Henry that no matter what his shortcomings at home, he had lived a good life and been a good father. Red evidently understood that—which is to say, he understood that Henry not only wanted him to go into the ministry; he needed him to. So Red went to seminary because he loved his father. His love was mixed with pity and, as he later acknowledged, with deep anger. But still he loved him. Moreover, it was in Red's bones to make the best, not the worst, of things, and it was in his bones and his religion to forgive. He never cherished wrongs. He and the entire family (including Henry) carried on very much as if Henry's anger and tyrannical behavior never happened. Certainly the correspondence is silent about it, except for the one acknowledgement (not apology) from Henry to Red, which never named the offense.

And despite Henry's behavior—which by rights should have driven

Red away from religion—Red continued to love the church. He loved it as an institution, as a tradition, and as a cultural experience. He loved the music, he loved the fellowship, he loved the little old ladies in periwinkle blue. He never felt superior to the church, never drifted away from it, and certainly never renounced it. He embraced it, even down to its fundamentalist language (of which he was a native speaker).

His homelife had been built around religion. Attending church, reading from the Bible, family devotionals morning and evening—all were central to Red's life growing up. He had never been allowed to miss church on Sunday and had never shown any inclination to. As a college student he had been a faithful member of the First Baptist Church in Bryan. His letters indicate that he continued to attend church regularly throughout his time in uniform; being away from home did not affect his churchgoing habits. When he was transferred to Germany, he became a full member of Central Baptist Church in Hillsboro. He assumed all the duties attendant on that dignity, including tithing and supporting building projects. Nevertheless, medicine appealed to Red Duke, and preaching did not.

When Red enrolled in seminary again, he was aware that even aside from making Henry happy and putting himself in a position to accomplish some good in the world, there were certain advantages to going down this path. There was not much question of whether he could make a go of medical school, but theology would obviously be easier. If preaching worked out, it would be a far less demanding profession than medicine, even though it paid less—a fact that he had ascertained in childhood by the direct route of asking. He would have more time to himself and to pursue his own interests than in any other profession. He would be treated with automatic deference and would have an entrée pretty much wherever he wanted to go.

And finally, Red already had a theatrical streak. This is evident even in family group photos. A touch of theatricality often runs through preachers, teachers, politicians—people who like to stand up before an audience and hold its attention by hook or by crook, but most gratifyingly, by force of personality. As a preacher, Red would not only get to perform; he would get to perform in the service of a higher good.

Red moved to Fort Worth to pick up where had left off at Southwestern Baptist Theological Seminary, a 1901 offshoot of Baylor's theological department. It sits on the highest hill in the county, now known as

Seminary Hill. "Surprisingly," Duke said, "for a guy that did not want to be there, I was really a good student. I liked to go to school and I loved history, archaeology, and languages." He studied Greek and Hebrew, and concurrently took classes in German at Texas Christian University (TCU). He had picked up some of the language while he was overseas and had developed an interest in it. He believed that "it's actually easier to take three languages at one time, because you are thinking linguistics."[2]

Fresh out of the army and living primarily on support from the GI Bill and his meager savings, Red had little money. He found a convenient room to rent at 3004 Ryan Avenue, just blocks from TCU and less than two miles north of the seminary. The owner, Mrs. James Robinson, was a widow who was delighted with her new tenant, a nice Texas boy attending seminary. Red would never forget Mrs. Robinson's kindness. On many an evening after a long day of classes on Seminary Hill, he made time to chat with her in her meticulously tended flower garden. That she had a son just out of medical school was of more than passing interest to Red. The more they talked, the more this second mother figure encouraged him not to give up on a career in medicine.[3]

At home, Red's parents still opposed medical school. But in Mrs. Robinson's garden he found steady assurance that the call of medicine could be just as powerful as the call of the church and that the two did not have to be mutually exclusive. His parents told him that he might not succeed in medical school, but making that argument, he said later, "was like throwing a piece of meat to my dog."[4] And he knew better.

Mrs. Robinson was not the only person encouraging Red to pursue medicine after seminary. There on the highest hill in Fort Worth in the library of Southwestern, he met—not, actually, for the first time—Betty Cowden. She was a pretty, petite brunette with fine, widely set eyes and a flawless complexion. She was sitting in the library at a table toward the back of the main room one day when Red strode in.

"I took notice, and he took notice," she told me. "I had known who he was because he came to Baylor. He was dating a Baylor girl in those last years at A&M, and he knew who I was because I was a friend of his girlfriend and was in that group of girls that he often ran into while in Waco. Neither one of us really knew each other, but we recognized each other immediately."

It was October of Red's first semester on campus. He struck up a conversation, invited Betty across the street for coffee, and then asked her to the state fair that weekend in Dallas. When Betty told her girl-friends about the date, they immediately set up a clamor. She couldn't go out with him, they said, because he went with "Mary Gene." Betty was having none of it. "'Well,'" she said, "'I don't know anything about that, but he has asked me, and I have said yes, and I am going.' I never did really know what that connection with Mary Gene had been except that I began to pick up little snippets here and there. They had met before he went into the service, and they wrote letters to each other, and she thought he was going to come home to marry her, and she and the Dukes formed a bond of friendship and love that I knew nothing about." Unapologetically she added, "I didn't even care about that."[5]

Soon Red was taking her to a party in Hillsboro to meet his friends, where she realized at once that she was being vetted. She passed mus-ter easily, but Red would have some much more intimidating muster to pass the next year, when Betty presented him for review by her parents.

Frances Elizabeth Cowden, Betty, was born in San Antonio on November 22, 1928. Six days earlier her future husband, Red Duke, had been born in Ennis on that cold, rainy night when his parents named him David and the nurse could not remember which mother was his.

For Betty Cowden home was Pearsall, Texas, about fifty miles south of San Antonio. Her father, George Cowden (1899–1963), was one of twelve siblings born to William Henry Cowden and Mary (Mamie) Sav-age. These paternal grandparents were known in the family as Gonga and Daddy Gonga. George, although he was the youngest of ten broth-ers, worked hard from his earliest age and was eventually put in charge of the Frio county ranch, one of three large ranches that his father owned.

George married Betty's mother, Frances Willard Coleman (1898–1988), in 1927. Betty, their first child, was followed by a son, George Malcolm, in 1930 and a daughter, Mary Jane, three years later. Daddy Gonga lived with his son George's family in his later years, and Betty recalls that the old man's preferences were not to be disputed: "I can remember my mother cooking biscuits on a wood-burning stove, the only way he would have them." Daddy Gonga had been very strict with his family of ten boys and two girls, and he was, Betty says, "very, very hard on my father. . . . Because my father grew up in what my mother called an 'angry family,' my mother insisted we were not going to have an angry family, and my father was in agreement. She taught us to say 'I love you' and we hugged each other at every opportunity. My brother and I, to this day, never end a conversation without 'I love you.'"[6]

Pearsall is a place where big ranches can be found covering vast miles of semi-arid brush country between San Antonio and the Rio Grande River. On this land the Cowdens ran cattle, and lots of them. It was scorchingly hot in the daytime in summer, and even the nights were warm. The night sky glittered with stars as far as you could see. This was not rich grassland country with open range, but mesquite and prickly pear cactus country where cattle and rancher alike had to be tough to survive. For hunters, it is big deer country, and it hosts other kinds of wildlife as well: coyotes, javelinas, coveys of bobwhite and blue quail, turkeys, roadrunners, and the ubiquitous and deadly diamond-back rattlesnake.

One of Betty's favorite photos of her father was taken after a long

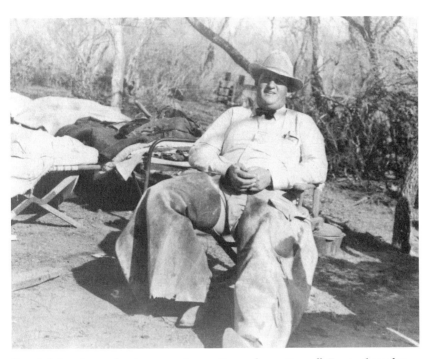

Betty's father, George Cowden, somewhere on the ranch near Pearsall, Texas, after a day working cattle.

day in the saddle somewhere in brush country on the ranch. His boots, chaps, and well-worn cowboy hat are dusty from miles of riding. His heavy denim shirt is no dress shirt. It is made to shield the wearer from the many hazards of working cattle in thick brush where every plant and insect has its own weaponry. An old cast-iron pot sits next to the campfire; two cots are scattered in the brush for the night's camp.

It is a scene right out of an old western. George Cowden offers a nod to the camera and a guarded smile. If you look at the photograph long enough, you notice an anomaly: he wears a bow tie with his cowboy gear to add a distinguished aristocratic tenor—for the name Cowden is known and highly regarded in Frio County. To no one who knew him, including Red, was he ever "George." He was "Mr. Cowden," a man who was big in stature and big in authority. He was treated with deference.

This was the world in which Betty grew up. When she was nine years old the family started moving into Pearsall for five days a week of the school year, but they returned to the ranch on weekends and during the summers. It is tempting to think of Betty as a cowgirl herself, adept at racing across the open range on horseback. She laughed at the notion. "Mother wanted my sister and me to be ladies," she said. "This was a working ranch and we did not ride horses for fun. My mother would not let me learn to milk a cow, because she said if you do not know how, you will never have to do it. She wanted me to be a lady, so she protected me."[7]

The Cowden siblings all went to Baylor in Waco. Betty noticed that when George Malcolm arrived on campus two years after she did, she suddenly stopped being Betty Cowden and started being George Cowden's sister—this in spite of the fact that she was well-known and well-liked by students and faculty alike. She was not annoyed; if anything, she was a little vain of her brother's quick success. George completed his law degree at Baylor and became a state representative in Austin (1963–66) as well as a trustee of the university. He retired to Austin, there to manage the family oil and gas royalties with the help of his son George III, also a Baylor law alumnus. Another of his four sons, Gordon, was a victim of the Aurora, Colorado, movie theater shooting in 2012.[8]

When Red Duke first met Betty he had no idea who these Cowdens were or even where Pearsall was, and the academic year would be over before he met them. But from the time they "took notice" at the library and went to the state fair together, Red and Betty were a couple. They dated all that academic year. Red never exactly proposed and Betty never exactly accepted; marriage simply came to be understood between them.[9]

During this courtship, Red continued to work diligently at Mrs. Robinson's on his bachelor of divinity—while he listened to her case in favor of medical school and drank in her steady encouragement. Betty, meanwhile, reinforced the landlady's advice.

At Texas A&M the influences on Red had been of a radically different kind. And his many activities, including the corps of cadets, football, yell leading, and general shenanigans, had cost him the grades that his parents had expected. Now, with his dormitory and barrack experiences behind him and an improved focus on good behavior that Southwestern, Mrs. Robinson, and Betty inspired, Red's grades shot up. He reported this triumph to Betty at the end his first school year (she had just finished her master's): "Received my grades yesterday. The cards were arranged in this order: Old Testament (O.T.), A; Greek, A; Social Ethics, A; Missions, A; Pastoral Ministry, A; and church History, B" (May 22, 1953).

At the end of the school year, Betty invited Red to see Pearsall and meet her family. The visit was a great success. Mr. Cowden and Red, both charismatic and both bigger than life, took to each other at once, in spite of the fact that Mr. Cowden had a long history of disliking his daughters' suitors. He made an exception for Red.

"He gave him a ride around the ranch," Betty said, "which would have taken hours." Although on the ranch they used horses to move cattle, for other purposes Mr. Cowden drove. He would roar around the ranch in his car, using it to take down brush where it was in the way or where he wanted a road. He used up a car in short order doing that. Additionally, he was a great sportsman and had hunted in exotic places—Africa, South America, Alaska. Red was bedazzled, and he and Mr. Cowden tore around the ranch in the increasingly battered car, cutting roads and talking cattle and hunting and fishing. They were entirely pleased with each other.[10]

Red recorded his impressions on the typewriter that had followed him from Texas A&M to Germany and back. His bread-and-butter letter to Betty after the visit has all the air of a moonstruck young man trying very hard to score points with the family. They would marry in December after that May meeting. And even before the wedding, Red and Betty had already made the mental move to a life in medicine rather than in preaching.

Betty planned the wedding from home in Pearsall; Red was still in Fort Worth studying. Letters back and forth between them plotted every detail of the preparations, including which typewriter they should keep—his or hers. Red resolved the question quickly: "If we keep a portable, it had best be mine" (November 22, 1953). It was a little harder to decide on china and pottery and the like, because Red's taste in colors and Betty's mother's were sometimes at odds.

As they fine-tuned the invitation list, Red realized that there would be more than two hundred guests. "I am ever staggered at the number," he wrote (October 27, 1953). On receiving their invitations, Red's friends took every opportunity to razz him. Andy Anderson, a relation of Monroe Dunaway Anderson of M. D. Anderson Cancer Center fame, promised to be there to help spring Red from his "apparent sentence of life imprisonment" and to study his plight so that he would not himself "be caught anytime soon" (November 25, 1953).

Red polished and repolished his old blue Ford. The task was more than a little frustrating. "The work I did yesterday had already oxidized by morning. Any other finish that I have ever worked with would be just about as you left it the day before. But not this one. I had to start all over and wax it as I polish[ed] it. Even now you can see the paint lose luster under the shiny coating of wax" (May 21, 1953). Red eventually made the car shine to perfection. But in the end he sold it for $600 to pay for Betty's wedding ring and borrowed another car for the wedding.

On December 18, 1953, Red and Betty were married in Pearsall at the First Baptist Church. It was a grand event in the small town. Sisters, best friends, and Betty's father performed their expected functions. Newspapers from Pearsall to Fort Worth reported the splendors of the seeded, pleated, entrained satin and lace gown of the bride, who was more perfect and more polished than even the elegant standards of the 1950s required.

Years earlier, Betty's father had taken the family to the Davis Mountains and Big Bend National Park. Betty loved the trip and promised herself that someday her honeymoon would be in that same wonderful

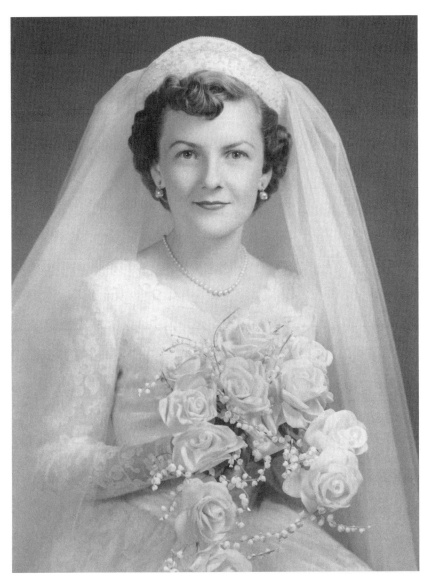

Betty Cowden on her wedding day, December 18, 1953.

place and at the same Indian Lodge, an adobe-style hotel built in the 1930s. The pancakes the couple ate for breakfast at the lodge were so good that Betty asked for the recipe. To this day, it is still the family recipe for pancakes.[11]

With the newlyweds settled impecuniously at 4024 Sandage in Fort

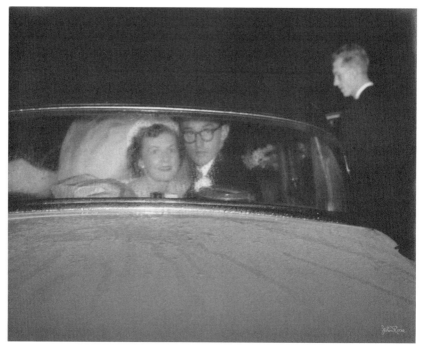

Mr. and Mrs. Red Duke pose for photos on a rainy wedding night in Pearsall, Texas, December 18, 1953.

Worth, Betty's parents drove up from Pearsall several times a year to deliver beef or venison from the ranch, and sometimes things more substantial, like a car that Mr. Cowden handed down to them to help out.[12] Once married, Red could not wait to get to Pearsall and the ranch to roam the outdoors and hunt deer with Mr. Cowden and Betty's brother George Malcolm. Over the years he and George Malcolm would go to the "high country," where Red was first introduced to big-game hunting in the mountains of British Columbia. In time, Colorado, Idaho, Alaska, Newfoundland, Afghanistan, and other places joined the list of Red's hunting grounds. He would develop a passion for big sky and rugged mountain hunts that helped motivate his commitment to preserving these places and their wildlife for future generations.

Red graduated from seminary in May of 1955. A young minister was expected to find a little country church to start with, and Red found one in Vaughn, not too far from Hillsboro, where he "supplied" while he was under consideration for full-time employment. This meant that he was trying out for the congregation, which would then decide whether or not to call him to its pulpit permanently. He discovered that he did not like writing two sermons a week, and the alternative was worse—going to a library of sermons, picking one out, and preaching it. "I was hell-bent on being original," he said. Evidently his efforts were appreciated. The church was on the verge of calling him when he was rescued by what he considered a divine intervention: "A tornado came through and tore the church down. So maybe it was like God speaking to me."[13]

And Red was prepared to listen. He had done what Henry wanted him to do. Now it was time to do what he wanted to do.

• • •

It is not entirely clear when Red Duke came under the influence of Albert Schweitzer (1875–1965). He wrote a paper on him in seminary. But Schweitzer was in the air, a household name, well before Red started seminary, and if he had not read Schweitzer before then, he would almost certainly have known who the great man was and what he had done. He could hardly have avoided knowing the name and basic narrative of the most admired person of the mid-twentieth century, who was to become his lifelong hero. He certainly patterned two important episodes of his life on Schweitzer's—his work in the Canadian outback and his two-year medical missionary work in Afghanistan. It is not beyond imagining that he could have patterned more than that on him. Even his seminary degree could owe something to Schweitzer, who was a preacher before he was a physician.

Schweitzer was a polymath whose accomplishments were staggering. He was not just a scholar, but a distinguished scholar in music, theology, and philosophy. He was a renowned concert organist who specialized in Bach. He held a licentiate in theology from the University of Strasbourg, where he lectured. In addition, he preached at St. Nicholas Church in Strasbourg, and he had a lifetime appointment as principal of the Theological College of St. Thomas, which was a part of the university.

But Schweitzer was a man who could not endure the thought of suffering, either human or animal, and he wanted to do something to relieve it—something direct, with his own hands. He saw an advertisement by the Paris Missionary Society for a physician in Gabon, a French colony in West Africa. To qualify for it he needed a medical degree. At the age of thirty, he resigned his comfortable position and enrolled as a medical student in the university where he had been teaching, with a specialty in tropical medicine. He completed his medical degree there at the age of thirty-eight. Then he packed up and in 1913 left for the remote jungle village of Lambaréné, Gabon.[14]

Schweitzer's friends, his family, his university, his church had been stunned when he set out at thirty to pursue a medical degree. But Red Duke, reading about him forty years later, was thrilled. The more he looked into Schweitzer's life, the more he liked what he saw.

Here was a man educated for the church and in possession of a lifetime benefice, determined to live a life of service. Yet Schweitzer was unfulfilled in his calling and asked of himself the same question Red was asking—is there more to doing good than preaching from a pulpit?

The conflicted Red Duke read Schweitzer's life story with eyes open wide.

CHAPTER 7

Canadian Outback

Red yearned for adventure—he wanted to meet new people in new places and pit himself against new obstacles. He also yearned to get busy doing good in the world. Like his hero Schweitzer, he was a missionary at heart with a superhuman abundance of energy and an unrelenting drive to make his life count for human betterment. If in the process he could prove himself morally, physically, intellectually, so much the better.

Moreover, he wanted to get started at once. Recognizing that he had but one available time slot, the summer of 1953, after his May graduation from seminary and before his December wedding, he told Betty of a plan he had made. "She should have known I was crazy right then," he said sixty years later.[1] It was a plan that caught his parents and friends by surprise, but Betty gamely supported him in it. She would stay at home in Pearsall planning the upcoming wedding, and Red would trek into the wilds of the Canadian outback to teach immigrant loggers English.

"My mother was really confused on hearing the news," Betty said, "and even asked if I was sure we were really engaged. I told her yes and not to be so concerned."[2] Besides, Betty knew Red well enough to know that nothing was going to stop him anyway. He was set on the outback, and the outback it would be.

This venture amounted to a postgraduate mission trip for the man who considered himself unproven and who was planning his future. In the *Saturday Evening Post* Red had come across a program that would send him into the Canadian wilderness as a teacher and laborer working with men who had immigrated to Canada for jobs in logging, mining, and laying railroad track. They included some of the toughest lumberjacks on earth. They were working in the remote northern wilderness, a place where harsh conditions and rough company would put Red's strength and determination to the test. It was exactly what he was looking for.

The adventure would be conducted under the auspices of Frontier College, a Canadian institution that was (and remains) dedicated to literacy. It was founded in 1899 by Alfred Fitzpatrick, with the purpose of improving the lot of an uneducated and illiterate or semiliterate labor force, native and immigrant. The work done by the men who were paid to log and mine and lay track was backbreaking and dangerous, and it was conducted under whatever conditions obtained—blistering heat, frigid cold, driving rain. The laborers it attracted were a rough, vigorous, profane lot—men willing to climb, top, and take down immense trees for ten hours a day, or to dig deep into mines, or lay track and drive great railroad spikes into it, and then to spend their nights in work camps where the food was as rough as they were and comforts were few.

Once the opportunity to fling himself at the Canadian wilderness had presented itself to Red, acting on it was simply a function of who and what he was. He had to do it. But the decision to spend two months in northern Canada a continent away from his bride-to-be in the summer before their wedding presaged other decisions Red would make in decades to come that would drip one-by-one into his marriage until they slowly but inexorably rusted it out.

George Cockburn, who joined the same program in the 1930s, wrote an essay about the job Duke was about to undertake. It was required reading for new employees on their way to the wilderness:

> For twenty summers I have watched the Labourer-Teachers of
> Frontier College at work in the far West of Canada—comfort-
> ing the needy in the distressful camps of the unemployed thir-
> ties, befriending the thousands of workers who stretched the
> great Alaska Highway through the Northern wilderness. . . . It
> is no easy thing for these young men who come from Canada's
> universities every summer to the bare, hard life of ten to
> twelve hours per day in manual labour under broiling sun or
> drenching rain. And after that they will be teaching for two
> or three hours a night: English, citizenship, and those things
> which will make better men out of their friends from Poland,
> Italy, and dozens of countries from whence comes Canada's
> newer blood.[3]

Red would have seen meaningful parallels between this Canadian opportunity and Albert Schweitzer's decampment to Africa. Like Schweitzer, Duke was going to a place where civilization was thin, to render aid to people who were hard to identify with and whose worthiness of the effort he was making could for that reason be doubted by many. (Duke at first feared he might doubt it himself. Schweitzer never did, and the strength of his conviction convinced the world.)

But there the similarities pretty much ended. Duke was making a trial run. Schweitzer didn't make trial runs; when he went into Africa, it was for life, and he burned bridges behind him. Duke was actually building bridges. And Canada for Duke, however much it was a testing ground, was also an adventure. It was never going to make him get his credentials in medicine and then go to Africa to practice invisibly in the jungle. That was not Red.

But there was nevertheless a very real connection between this Canadian adventure and the two years that he would later spend in the Middle East as a medical missionary. It proofed him against any inertia that might have kept him from taking the plunge into service. And it set him up emotionally for real sacrifice in Afghanistan. Red was playful, but Canada was not just play. It was for real.

When Duke reached camp on June 19, he wrote his first letter to Betty. He had brought along his well-pounded typewriter for the trip, but this letter is handwritten and more introspective than usual:

> Contrary to what is probably common belief, I am in fine
> condition and have encountered no falling trees or savage
> bears. . . . I have tromped through a lot of "bush" country
> as they call it. The appearance of the country is just as the
> pictures indicate; trees, rocks, and lakes with small islands in
> them. I am some 792 miles from Toronto. I arrived yesterday
> afternoon in Huron Bay. . . .
>
> The most important thing that I can learn from the
> experience that the College has put ahead of me is to go in
> among these men and become such a part of them that they
> will feel I am a part of them. That is very very difficult for
> me because I am so human that I am greatly influenced by
> outward appearances. Here is a situation where humility and

love are mandatory. I hope I can always keep the facts before
me because my ability to help them depends directly upon this
fact. (July 26, 1953)

It is somewhat surprising that Duke expected to have to teach himself
to identify with the loggers whose company he found himself in. But he
was soon reporting how intelligent they were, and that some of them
spoke four or five languages. And the camp itself was more civilized
than he had expected it to be:

> They say that this is a model bush camp. In all truth, the camp
> is much nicer than I had expected. They have showers and flush
> toilets that are a rarity in most camps. To give you an idea of
> the different kind of fellows that I will have, we have French,
> French-Canadian, German, Yugoslav, Czech, Rumanian, Bul-
> garian, Italian, Latvian, and Swiss. It would break your heart to
> see the life these fellows lead. They work hard, real hard, all day.
> The average man cuts and stacks two cords of pulp wood every
> day. We get up at 5:30 and have breakfast at 6:00. Most of them
> are gone at 6:30. They come in a few minutes before lunch and
> are back out again til dinner. (June 28, 1953)

With his sympathies already engaged, Red was not likely to fail at identifying with his students. When Alfred Fitzpatrick had conceived the idea
of Frontier College, central to it was the notion of the laborer/teacher
who commands the respect of his students by demonstrating respect for
them and the work they do and by being able to do it himself. He was a
man of democratic principles who believed in the equality of work done
by the mind and that done by the body. He sought not just to make the
student more like the teacher, but to make the teacher like the student.
Teachers were to labor alongside their students during the day, and
teach them at night. "Nothing but efficiency appeals to these men—efficiency, not in mathematics or literature, or theology, but in actual labor
of the hands, and in their particular brand of manual labor."[4]

"My first job," Red reported home to Hillsboro, "was the assistant
to the bull cook. The bull cook is the general handyman or janitor
for the camp. The particular bull cook that we have here is a little old

Frenchman. That rascal can really get after it too. He ran my rear off trying to get things done that he wanted done. On Tuesday morning we swept, washed, scrubbed, ran a rubber dryer over the floor, and mopped it. This happens once a week." The most pleasant job dispensed by the bull cook was "carrying the garbage in a sled drawn by two horses to the dump."

Red's earnest hope that his next assignment would not be with the bull cook was fulfilled; instead he was set to stamping wood. Companies must stamp their wood, he explained, just as ranchers brand their cattle "We use a hammer with a large 'O.P.' on it," he said. "This is a nice job except the wrists are not quite accustomed to it and the hammering on the end of the logs drives more black flies out of the wood." But Red's main form of manual labor was felling trees.

The Toronto offices of Frontier College required a daily log, and Red turned in a carefully typed report at summer's end, emphasizing the teaching, not the logging, part of his duties. He saved a copy. Selected entries provide a snapshot of his activities:

> June 22—I arrived at Camp 53 and was given the temporary task of splitting logs for firewood. I met two Yugoslavs and six Germans. All of these men expressed some desire to learn English. I hope that I am not moving too fast. One just seems to fall into discussion of English. We also spent about one hour talking about the geography and the ways of life on the North American continent. Most of the questions were directed to Texas I must admit.
> June 24—I began my first favor for one of the men. I started filling out an accident form for Oswald Peterlik.
> June 26—I am very impressed with the cooperation of the company. They gave me a set of horseshoes today and the material to build the boxes. I finished the boxes in the evening.
> June 29—The first step was taken in the organization of the English classes. I divided the group into two sections, the RED and the BLUE.
> July 4—We had good informal discussions. Four men: Joe Liska, Amile, Stan Srbek (Czechs) and Ludwig Udonic

talked about some of the confusing and difficult problems in the English language.

July 9—I had a very interesting discussion with a man, a very peculiar man, concerning the various systems of government. He has developed a theory and a plan that all may live together in the world in peace and harmony when there are more dictatorships.

July 11—Today we had a very good discussion of the science of photography. Four Germans and a Latvian as well as a Polish fellow participated. Where English was not understood, they all understood the science of figures and numbers.

July 19—I had a very good talk with a man named Kruze from Latvia. For a while we talked languages. Then we had a fine discussion on the two major systems of measurements.

We had a fine participation for about an hour and a half on European football. This is the best percentage of participation yet.[5]

One day a small forest fire flared up near camp. Red leaped into action with the others and helped extinguish it. He did not actually go out with the men all day every day—he had found that keeping up with the best of the best lumberjacks in the world could be exhausting. On the evenings after the days when he had done a really respectable job of logging, he would often be too tired to write Betty. But many other nights, after cutting trees and teaching, he would while away what was left of his waking time by recounting his adventures to her, recalling the bears and moose and other animals he had seen, and perhaps bragging just a little.

Shortly after he arrived in Canada, Red had received a letter from his maternal grandfather, Ivo. Papa, the retired railroad man, minced no words. He had important things on his mind:

[June 19, 1953]
  My dear grandson:
  That was nice of you to run off and not come by so that we could have a little talk. When I got your dad's letter telling me where you had gone I was surprised as I had a question that is not clear in my mind and I am going to ask you for your opinion. I have known for some time you cannot make up your mind fully as to what you want to do. I have been wondering which is the best, a contented mind or more education? Will you please give me your opinion? I am waiting your return so that we can talk Sony. May God help and bless you. Papa.

Ivo was very good at stirring the pot, Red knew. Another note Ivo sent his grandson upon hearing about the December wedding plans was a simple index card carefully typed and centered—food for thought from grandfather to grandson:

  a thought—
  Marriage never fails but
  Participants can and do . . .
  Think it over
  Papa

Whether Ivo intended this message as a general warning for the future or a specific comment on Red's then-current occupation is open to question.

In spite of all the family advice, including the constant nudging of his father to find a home behind the pulpit, Red made up his own mind. What was best for Red Duke was both a contented mind *and* more education.

It had been a summer of discovery. Frontier College had liked his work so much that they asked if he would take a winter assignment.[6] Red politely declined. He headed home—and to Betty—by train.

CHAPTER 8
Medical School Days

James Duke—Red Duke—was a sparkling medical student, full of enthusiasm and verve. This was combined with an excellent command of medicine. He could apply those assets to patient care and capture the loyalty of his patients and their confidence in his ability to care for them. The combination of enthusiasm and insight made Red Duke an outstanding physician

—DONALD W. SELDIN, MD

"It was the most awful color as the sky went dark," Betty said some six decades later of the clouds over Dallas on the afternoon of Tuesday, April 2, 1957. She and Red had been married three years, and Red was now a freshman medical student at UT Southwestern in Dallas. They lived in a second-floor apartment with a view across Stemmons Freeway, which led to the new Southwestern medical campus several miles south off Harry Hines Boulevard.

> It was late afternoon and I had been shopping. When I saw the sky turn dark green I raced back to the apartment and watched out the kitchen window as an immense tornado swept down the freeway headed directly for the medical school. Red was there, and an awful feeling of dread came over me. I feared I might never see him again. Thankfully he made it home later that night with tales of racing to a nearby cement culvert where he took refuge with several of his classmates and watched as the tornado approached and swirled away at the last moment.[1]

Red was squeezed inside the culvert and squinting upward at the sky as rain pelted his face and the tornado raged nearby. "Tornado Slashes Wide Path of Death and Destruction," read the next morning's *Dallas*

Times Herald headline. Ten died that evening, and hundreds of others were injured.[2] Next to the medical school at Parkland Hospital, more than 176 of the injured were cared for. Local newspapers praised the emergency planning and efficiency of the school's faculty and residents, who labored late into the night saving lives. Red, a freshman medical student standing on the sidelines, caught an exhilarating glimpse of his future self also saving lives in the midst of chaos. He was hooked, and he longed for the day when he could be in the thick of the action.

While Red had taken the tornado that had struck his church several years before as a sign that the pulpit was not his calling, this tornado told him that he was in the right place at the right time. For him, it was a divine affirmation that as a physician he could do things for humanity that a preacher could not.

Red had made the switch from graduate seminarian to freshman medical student two years previously, in the summer of 1955. One blistering hot day he had found himself standing on the roof of a house in Fort Worth. He was a recently ordained minister questioning his future in the church. He and his bride had been married more than a year, and on this particular day he was working a construction job for extra money to take Betty on a wild and open trip to Alaska. As he stood on that scorching roof dreaming of Alaskan glaciers and rivers thick with salmon, he knew that there was unfinished business at hand. The harder he pounded nails into shingles, the more he felt it. The unfinished business was medical school. "Finally I said to myself, 'Well, Lord, I can't get this out of my system. Is this what I am supposed to do, or are we going to find out?' I got down off that roof and went over to TCU. That was in the summer of 1955. I had gotten enough courses out of the way to start school in Dallas at Southwestern in 1956. I even took some stuff over just to work at it. I made real good grades."[3]

Red's premedical studies and grades paid off; he was accepted into medical school at UT Southwestern in the fall of 1956. Registration took place September 5–8.[4] Red and Betty moved from their apartment in Fort Worth near Seminary Hill to a Dallas apartment not far from Love Field and an easy drive to Southwestern. Betty had taught first grade in Fort Worth; she taught third grade in Dallas. Her new school took her into the west side of the city in one of its poorest neighborhoods, near Singleton Boulevard, the same neighborhood where Clyde

Barrow of Bonnie and Clyde fame had grown up. Red began his medical studies in a much better part of town, where the University of Texas Southwestern Medical School was growing by leaps and bounds—a far cry from the school's early beginnings.

When Baylor University's medical school moved from Dallas to Houston in 1943, half the squabbling medical faculty remained in Dallas to become the Southwestern Medical School of the University of Texas; the other half went on to Houston with Baylor and their dean, Walter Moursund. In 1949, the medical school still in Dallas affiliated with the University of Texas. It originally began as a collection of World War I military barracks. These were intended to be replaced within five years, but instead limped along more than fourteen. Located at Oak Lawn and Maple Avenues, the school was adjacent to Parkland Hospital, which first opened in 1894 on what was then a seventeen-acre wooded site. The hospital was named Parkland because the land had originally been purchased for a city park.[5]

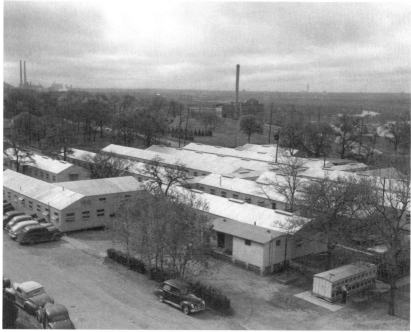

"The Shacks," early home of Southwestern Medical School in the late 1940s. Courtesy of UT Southwestern Archives.

Students and faculty referred to the maze of dilapidated military buildings that made up UT's new medical school as "the Shacks." The architecture, they observed, could best be described as "henhouse classic." Early alumni reported cold winters when the cadavers froze; gross anatomy class was postponed until the thaw. Research during the hot summer months was difficult for lack of air conditioning. And funding for permanent buildings was not forthcoming from the Texas legislature. The Southwestern Medical Foundation appealed for state support repeatedly and at the end of 1951 finally succeeded in getting Texas governor Allan Shivers to lead a delegation from Austin to Dallas to determine whether the legislature should appropriate funds for permanent buildings.

As recorded in the Southwestern Medical Foundation publication 75 Years of Vision, a pathologist recalled that "students, fellows and faculty were lined up in the shacks to welcome the governor and his entourage. The governor walked in through the back of one of the long shacks, and as he got halfway down the edifice, a window simply dropped out of the wall. The governor continued walking and another thirty yards later, one of his feet went through the floor. We knew from the look on his face that he was going to help us."[6]

In 1952 the Texas legislature approved $2.75 million for a new basic sciences building on a new campus several miles away off Harry Hines Boulevard and just two miles from downtown Dallas.[7] Parkland Hospital broke ground on the new campus that same year, and in 1954 the Texas legislature appropriated $3.5 million for a new clinical sciences building.[8] What was once a collection of military shacks was now a fast-growing medical center that would never return to the days of frozen cadavers and mass faculty departures, which for many months in the early 1950s outdistanced recruitment.

These events were significant to Red Duke's medical future as he registered for his freshman year on September 5, 1956. For UT Southwestern, the new facilities would usher in tremendous growth and the recruitment of outstanding faculty who would build educational and Nobel-class research programs that remain today a hallmark of UT Southwestern.

On January 29, 1955, the new Basic Science Hall (renamed the Edward H. Cary Basic Science Hall in 1960) opened on the new medical campus adjacent to the new Parkland Hospital, which had also moved from the Shacks off Oak Lawn Avenue to open in 1954.[9] The new Parkland, with its gleaming operating suites and trauma rooms, would provide top-notch training facilities and equipment for students like Red Duke for years to come. As the new basic science building opened, research faculty and students alike thankfully relocated from the Shacks.

• • •

The academic year was divided into three terms of twelve weeks, making twelve terms over the next four years. This would provide the training required for the degree of doctor of medicine. Class size was one hundred, and tuition for the first year was all of three hundred dollars. Books and supplies were estimated by the school administration to cost another three hundred. Red, pinching every penny that the young couple earned, discovered that he would be required to provide his own microscope, with Bausch and Lomb, American Optical, Zeiss, or Leitz brands recommended (carrying case required).[10] Thanks to Red's military service, however, the cost of most of his medical education was covered. Betty was teaching, and both families helped out during these lean years. Even Henry was helpful now that medical school had become a fact.

Red's first two years of study would thankfully be in the new basic sciences building on the new campus. Juniors and seniors would still be meeting in the Shacks. Plans for a new clinical building were underway. Here Red bonded with his fellow students as they dove into first-year required courses, which included biochemistry, biophysics, gross anatomy, histology-embryology, neuroanatomy and physiology, physical medicine, and psychiatry.[11]

The volume and density of the content facing medical students was formidable, and Red's schedule was jam-packed throughout the four years of twelve-week blocks. Moreover, scheduled classes in gross anatomy, psychiatry, and biochemistry alternated by term between weekday and Saturday scheduling.

Having grown up hunting and fishing, Red did not, upon meeting his cadaver, find that his knees buckled. Such was not the case with some of his classmates. Gross anatomy is considered a rite of passage

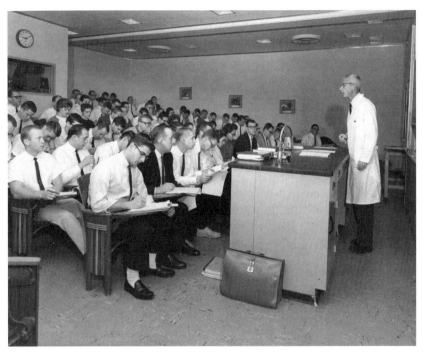

Dr. Robert M. Price teaching microbiology at Southwestern Medical School in the mid-1950s on the new Harry Hines campus. White shirts and ties were the look of the day, with ties removed for gross anatomy. Image courtesy of UT Southwestern Archives.

that every medical student must face. Red was eager to learn, and if he was uneasy with his first cut of the scalpel into human flesh, he certainly wasn't going to show it. Additionally, having gone through the army and seminary, he was several years older than most of his classmates. He projected an air of confidence and maturity, even if he had at first sometimes wondered how he would stack up against his younger peers straight out of pre-med college preparation.

Betty believed that Red worked all the harder because Henry, in promoting seminary, had repeatedly warned him that he did not have the scholastic chops for medical school. But he did have the chops. "He was like a sponge," Betty said, "absorbing everything that came his way. He simply loved medical school and was determined not to fail."[12] Red has his own more colorful way of making that point. "Once I got into medical school," he said, "I was just as happy as a pig in slop."[13] Staying at school late, camped out in the library and typically studying alone rather than in groups, he applied the work ethic his father had insisted upon. "I wasn't the smartest guy in the class," he would say, "but the others did not work as hard as I did."

Rarely did he study around the apartment, recalls Betty, especially after they started a family during his junior year. For the most part, his student life was centered on the new Southwestern campus and affiliated hospitals. He returned home late most days during the first four years of medical school, and later yet during his residency. He was always home well after dark.

While the deadly Dallas tornado certainly got his attention in April of his first year, another event three months earlier, on January 30, 1957, had shaken the entire medical school. Second-year student Paul Pendergraft was killed shortly after eight o'clock in the morning on his way to school. Red and his freshman classmates had scarcely arrived for neuroanatomy when Pendergraft's 1949-model sedan collided just blocks away with a big, six-wheel truck carrying eleven thousand pounds of produce.[14] Pendergraft suffered severe head injuries and was pronounced dead on arrival next door at Parkland. Red and his classmates tried to make sense of such a tragic loss so close to home. Medical students—physicians—were supposed to be invincible. Pendergraft was just twenty-three, five years younger than Red on that day.

The loss of a fellow student sent a reminder though the school that life is short and that every single day must be lived to the hilt. As soon as he had taken his last first-year exam on June 5, Red took the money he had saved by roofing houses, bought a new Ford ranch wagon, and headed north with Betty for a summer in Alaska. It would be a trip neither would ever forget. It was a time before children, when they could travel and explore at will, while they were still young and carefree, and not enough life had accumulated around them to create many complications.

When they returned, Betty announced that it was time to start a family. Hank, the first of four children, was born the following year, on June 30, 1958. Another big change occurred as Red's second year of medical school began. Betty's father, Mr. Cowden, helped them buy a small, three-bedroom house at 3616 Valley Ridge Road, just six miles from the Southwestern campus; the drive took only minutes in the early mornings before rush hour.

This was the young couple's first home with room enough to entertain. They welcomed the additional space, and many a weekend they hosted their friends from both seminary in Fort Worth and medical school in Dallas. It made for an interesting meeting of minds as their friends coming from different world views hashed over a potpourri of social and medical issues. Red, the social animal he was, loved these encounters and often served as the ringleader, stirring the pot to bring up all the possible bones of contention.

The fare at these dinner parties was typically Mexican dishes that Betty and Red had perfected over the years. Betty's crispy tacos were the specialty of the house, and her nachos and burritos were much in demand. But not everyone took a fancy to such fiery concoctions. Recalls Betty, "One of my best friends from seminary, who was my brother's roommate at Baylor, used to douse his plate with ketchup. I'll never forget how Red and I laughed and gave him a hard time."[15]

As a medical student at UT Southwestern, the former Aggie yell leader and credentialed Baptist preacher was now also a University of Texas Longhorn. Red's friends from A&M and seminary needled him gleefully, demanding to know how an Aggie yell leader and preacher could ever let himself become a Longhorn. Red, without missing a beat, replied piously: "I'm just being a good missionary." Often Red took center stage, talking about medicine and sometimes controversial social issues that raised the eyebrows of the seminary friends, one of whom once responded, "Red, your church veneer is starting to slip."[16]

Red's sophomore schedule was as well stuffed as ever, except for a little more free time on Saturdays. As they had during the first year, classes started at eight in the morning and ran until four. Second-year coursework included physiology, pharmacology, microbiology, clinical pathology, introduction to medicine, psychology, preventive medicine, and physical medicine.[17]

By the third year Red would be in the classroom and laboratory less and into the clinical setting more. This was the beginning of his clinical years, with their focus on patient care. The new Southwestern campus continued to grow, and Dean A. J. Gill was deeply gratified by the quality of the education and patient care his school now offered. At UT in Austin the new Dallas medical school was featured on February 15, 1959, in the campus newspaper, *The Daily Texan*. Red was now rotating through a variety of clinical experiences as part of the third-year curriculum. Kay Ponder's reporting provides a look into a medical student's world at this time.

> The 400 students receive instruction from a full-time faculty of 91 supplemented by the part-time services of more than 600 Dallas specialists. . . . These specialists, teaching the juniors and seniors, give depth and breadth to the program while the regular faculty give it continuity. Dr. A. J. Gill, Dean of Southwestern Medical School, says, "It's like owning an organ with 100 keys. You won't need every key to play every tune, but when you need to hit that one certain note, the key is there."
> . . . Having an acceptance rate of 1 out of 5, the caliber of students is high, as the work would "stagger a weak student."
> The juniors and seniors step outside the classroom, sporting the traditional white jacket, and move into various hospitals and clinics. This is the clinical science curriculum where the student first becomes acquainted with the day-to-day problems [of patients]. . . . Dean Gill describes the quantity and variation in patients as "unbelievable."[18]

Red not only excelled in medical school; he exceeded his own expectations. As an undergraduate he had sacrificed his grades to his social life, but a married Red Duke focused entirely on mastering medicine. Most students who are choosing between internal medicine and surgery pick one or the other. Red Duke picked both. Four key medical mentors were decisive in this dual focus, which shaped his future. They were Donald Seldin, Tom Shires, Stanley Dudrick, and Robert Shaw.

• • •

Donald W. Seldin (b. 1920), of UT Southwestern, is a man to whom Red assigned much of the credit for his successes. "The real brains behind Southwestern," he said, "is a guy named Don Seldin. That man is smart and a real hero of mine. He liked me, and I did a straight medicine internship with him, as had a couple of other guys that were surgeons up there not much older than me. He is why Southwestern exists. I did a straight medicine internship with him because I love medicine. A good surgeon is a fairly good internist . . . otherwise he is just going to be a technician. There is a whole lot more to being a good surgeon than operating."[19]

Seldin has been called the intellectual father of UT Southwestern, and he was a medical father figure for Red Duke throughout Duke's undergraduate and postgraduate years. What Seldin gave Duke was an appreciation for the relationship between internal medicine and superiority in surgery. Duke echoed a sentiment that he had learned early on from Seldin when he said that if a surgeon is not a good internist, "he is just going to be a technician. There is a whole lot more to being a good surgeon than operating." Duke believed like Seldin that surgery is ideally supported by a strong background in the integrated approach that a good internist brings to the bedside. Seldin was also a stickler for patient-centric care supported by rigorous research, and through his example Duke developed the necessary research interest and broad medical focus to be a triple hitter who could teach, treat patients, and conduct research.

Seldin first arrived at UT Southwestern in 1951, in the very early days of the old campus just months before Governor Shivers walked through an army barracks with falling windows and uncertain floors. A Yale-trained physician, Seldin had completed his residency in internal medicine in New Haven and was a Yale faculty member from 1944 to 1951, when the new UT Southwestern Medical School asked him to come to Texas. Faculty at the time were fleeing the school in droves.[20] Within a year after his arrival in Dallas, Seldin was named chairman of internal medicine, and he served in that position for thirty-five years, from 1952 to 1988. On March 16, just five months before Red's death, Seldin Plaza was dedicated at Southwestern, honoring the intellectual father of the medical school with a bronze statue.[21] Red was too ill to attend.

During his tenure, Seldin elevated research and recruited and trained outstanding students whom he would then send off for advanced training and recruit back to fill key faculty positions. During the Seldin years, UT Southwestern produced four Nobel laureates in physiology or medicine and ten members of the Institute of Medicine or the National Academy of Sciences. Many of these honors were directly attributable to Seldin's insightful recruitment and career guidance.[22]

Looking back on his mentor's influence, Red recalled, "When the first two men up there got a Nobel Prize, I wrote him and told him, I said,

'You ought to be getting this,' because he was just one of these incredible figures in medicine." He added, "He never took his boards because he did not think anybody could examine him."[23]

Seldin was a great wit. In 1988, when he retired from the chairmanship of internal medicine in Dallas to become chair emeritus, his former students collected some of their chief's renowned words of wisdom[24]—words that Red remembered for a lifetime and sometimes used on his own students:

Here's a dime. Go call your mother. She will know the answer to my question. Tell her that you're coming home.

Education is what you have left after you have forgotten the facts.

Education does not change personalities—it simply makes them more difficult to deal with.

This is a beautiful example of therapeutic frenzy combined with abysmal ignorance.

From Seldin, Red learned how to be a well-rounded, patient-centered physician with a big-picture grasp of physiology and systems that he could marry to his surgical skills and research interests. That Seldin had been a risk taker and put his career on the line to migrate from Yale to a medical school composed of a few rundown army barracks next to a railroad track spoke to Red, in spite of the fact that when he took the job at long distance Seldin had no clue what he was getting into. Seldin's story about his first trip to Dallas (back when Red was graduating from A&M) is preserved in his own words as part of a Southwestern oral history project:

> I never visited Dallas prior to accepting the position. It's incredible. These days nobody ever accepts a job until after several visits and major offers. . . . I arrived in Dallas on January 8, 1951. At the corner of Maple Avenue and Oak Lawn was a filling station. My wife, daughter, and I had driven from New Haven. I wanted to see the medical school before we

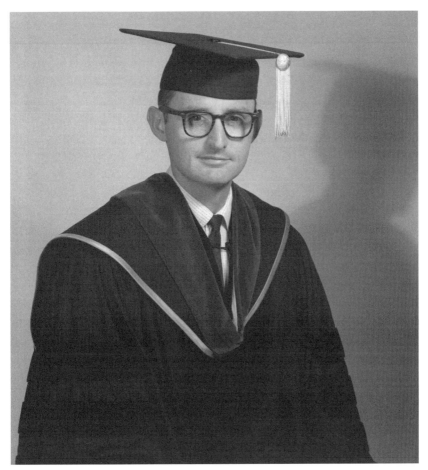

James Henry "Red" Duke Jr., MD. Graduation day, May 30, 1960. Courtesy of UT Southwestern Archives.

settled anywhere. I asked the filling station attendant where the medical school was. He gestured in the direction of the railroad tracks down the street. I drove the car there. I looked around and saw nothing. I came back and told the attendant that I had not seen a medical school, only shacks and garbage. "That's it," he said.[25]

For Red Duke this was an important story, an assurance that sometimes you have to take risks, go places others might not go, and apply yourself

to making something great where once there was little. It was a lesson he would act on himself. But first he needed to graduate, and he
did that on May 30, 1960, when he and ninety-nine of his classmates
received their medical diplomas. In this class of one hundred, only two
were women—Peggy Joann Dyer and Thelma Marie Smith.[26] Twelve
students, including Red, were matched to remain at Southwestern to
continue their residency training at Parkland in various fields.[27] For
Red, it would be general surgery. Now, as a resident in surgical training,
he came to know three additional mentors. They took center stage in
his life and helped shape his trajectory as a surgeon.

• • •

George Thomas Shires (1925–2007) was a graduate of UT Southwestern who had completed his residency at Parkland. As Red was
graduating from A&M in 1950, Shires had just completed additional
training at the US Naval Medical Research Institute in Bethesda.
Shires's distinguished service as a surgeon on the navy hospital vessel
USS *Haven* furthered his advancement to academic medicine, and in
1957 he joined the faculty of UT Southwestern. In 1961 he was named
chairman of the Department of Surgery just as Red was beginning his
residency.[28]

Shires was somewhat reserved for Duke's taste and had little sense
of humor. Those traits did not appeal to him, but he was there to learn,
and Shires had much to teach. To begin with, he was working with the
Dallas Fire Department to initiate one of the country's earliest paramedic systems. "You have to remember," said Duke, "in those days if
you got into an accident, there were no paramedics or well-equipped
vehicles to get you to the emergency room. In Dallas you came by car,
perhaps the back of a police car, or commonly in the back seat of a
local taxi. Taxis in those days had plastic seats so they could transport
patients and wipe the blood off the seat for the next fare."[29] Thanks to
Shires, Duke acquired a familiarity with paramedicine that was useful
to him a decade later as he worked with the Houston Fire Department
to organize paramedic systems and his air ambulance program.

Shires's research in the early 1960s on the physiology of shock
also interested Duke. Going against the practice of the time, Shires
demonstrated through his research that surgical patients and patients
with other trauma need intravenous saline solution. This was game-
changing medicine, and exposure to academic surgeons like Shires who

combined research and surgical practice to improve patient outcomes had a profound impact on Red Duke's career.

Shires's interest in establishing trauma and burn centers was another area that Duke learned from and applied in the years ahead. Since severe burn patients burn more calories in repair each day than they can take in, developing a way to feed them intravenously was a major area of research at the time. Burn patients requiring surgery, or patients unable to take in food by mouth, stood little chance until a way could be found to meet their nutritional needs through intravenous methods.

• • •

Stanley J. Dudrick (b. 1935) was a young surgical resident at the University of Pennsylvania who in the early 1960s took on the challenge of feeding patients who could not eat. In years to come, this same Dudrick would play a pivotal role in Red's surgical career. Dudrick's mentor as a student had been a towering figure in surgery, Jonathan Rhoads. One day after losing three surgical patients during a weekend on call, a distraught Dudrick announced to Rhoads that he was seriously considering leaving surgery; he could not bear to lose patients after skillfully performed, complex operations followed by intensive postoperative care. Rhoads confided in Dudrick that he was seeing the most difficult cases referred to the department, because no one else could help them. Many of the patients were manifestly not strong enough to withstand the stress of the surgeries they needed to live. What was needed was a way to feed these patients intravenously and build their strength before sending them into surgery.

Then, recalls Dudrick, Rhoads hurt him with words that would change his life. Said Rhoads, "Stan, if you want to be a quitter, go ahead. But at least give a year or so to help solve the critical nutritional deficiencies and find a way to feed and strengthen these patients so they have a fighting chance to survive the surgery." Dudrick accepted the challenge.[30]

While small molecules like carbohydrates, minerals, and vitamins posed little problem for intravenous feeding, administering larger molecules like protein and fat intravenously posed a major obstacle and was one of the bigger research problems of the day. The technology to break proteins down into their component amino acids for intravenous infusion was still being researched.

Dudrick worked night and day with beagle puppies to perfect total feeding by intravenous means and to demonstrate that it could sustain and save lives. The puppies were fed exclusively by a tube inserted into a large central vein near the heart. They grew and developed normally via Dudrick's improved intravenous feeding technique, then referred to most commonly as intravenous hyperalimentation.

Dudrick was tireless in caring for his canine patients. Even his family got involved, with his children visiting the puppies on nights and weekends and his wife sewing custom harnesses to make the intravenous tubes more comfortable. Dudrick added other apparatus that delivered each puppy's entire food intake. In time, his intravenously fed puppies rivaled their orally fed twin siblings in growth and vigor. His technology and infusion techniques maintained caloric and nutritional balance using the intravenous route alone. After he had demonstrated that his approach worked in dogs, he went on to demonstrate that it worked in human patients, too.[31]

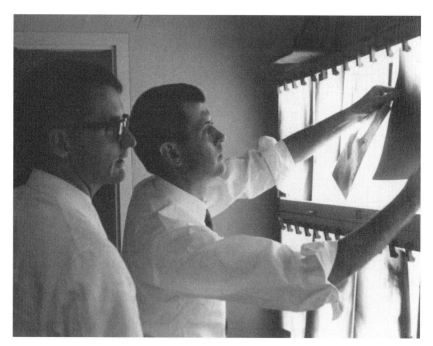

Red Duke (left) reviewing patient X-rays with Jack Reynolds, a radiologist at UT Southwestern during the mid-1960s.

Total intravenous hyperalimentation, more commonly known today as total parenteral nutrition (TPN), was born. Today TPN is used in hospitals worldwide to boost caloric intake and feed patients who otherwise would likely die, and who could certainly not tolerate complex medical interventions, including surgery and cancer treatments like chemotherapy and radiation therapy. For severely burned patients, infants born prematurely and/or without functioning alimentary tracts, cancer patients, and patients with severe malnutrition from any cause, the procedure is a fixture in modern health care.

Dudrick was renowned for both research and surgical skills. He was in demand to present his findings at conferences and medical schools around the country and the world. That was how he came to visit Tom Shires and his research team in Dallas. There in the back of the room, Dudrick remembers seeing a tall, thin redhead with brown eyes, wearing a white shirt and plaid tie. With black horn-rimmed glasses and short hair, Red's look was more like Buddy Holly's than it was like his cowboy persona of years to come. Looks aside, Red Duke was listening quietly, with great interest.

Within a year, Duke would meet Dudrick again, this time at an annual senior surgery resident's conference at the University of Wisconsin. Duke was intrigued by Dudrick's nutritional research, and he determined to develop his skills in that area to become not just a good general surgeon, but a good academic surgeon. The meetings with Stan Dudrick would prove fortunate for Duke and Dudrick both, as their future paths would cross in surprising ways.

Thus directly and indirectly, Tom Shires, Red Duke's chairman of surgery in Dallas, influenced his career. The newly minted Dr. Duke took to heart everything that he observed, and in Shires he observed a dedicated academic surgeon whose work ethic he admired hugely. He might find Shires's style rigid and formal, but in substance, here was a man who got things done and looked to the future for innovative solutions to current problems.

• • •

Robert R. Shaw (1905–1992), a 1933 graduate of the University of Michigan's School of Medicine, was one of the first thoracic surgeons in the Dallas area during the early 1960s. He began his private practice in Dallas in 1938 and practiced continuously in the area with the exception of two diversions: the first for World War II service in the Medical Corps of the army in the European theater, and the second for volunteer service with MEDICO from December 1961 to June 1963, when he assisted at the Avicenna Hospital in Kabul, Afghanistan.[32] As a first-year medical student meeting members of the faculty, Duke took an instant liking to Shaw. Duke considered him "one of the most interesting and dynamic faculty members we had. That he was a talented surgeon, a great teacher, and someone who took the time to volunteer his skills to help other countries was really impressive and memorable to me."[33]

MEDICO had been started by Tom Dooley, a young physician who in the late 1950s established a jungle clinic in Laos and with donated supplies treated people who had never seen a doctor. He called for medical educators "to arouse in your students a sense of duty to all men." John F. Kennedy cited MEDICO as one inspiration for the creation of the Peace Corps.[34] Tom Dooley met an untimely death from cancer in 1961 at the age of thirty-four, but his example mobilized physicians like Robert Shaw to take their medical know-how afar. Shaw took his to a hot, dusty hospital in Afghanistan, where he would return again and again to help the desperately needy in a country where he was at first the only heart surgeon. He performed surgeries, trained other surgeons, and brought some of them to Dallas for advanced training that was not possible in Afghanistan.

On September 1, 1961, Shaw returned to Dallas and UT Southwestern, where he was named professor of thoracic surgery and chairman of the Division of Thoracic Surgery. The timing could not have been better for Red Duke, who was beginning his graduate training in surgery and looked forward to working with Shaw on his thoracic service. Not only was he eager to learn from Shaw; he was also spellbound by the stories Shaw brought back to Dallas from his travels, especially in Afghanistan.

Duke worked long hours beside Shaw to meet the endless surgical needs that a busy county hospital like Parkland provided around the clock. Gunshot wounds were among the common procedures the two attended. Red was struck by a remark of Shaw's one day as they successfully tracked a bullet that stopped just millimeters short of a patient's heart. As Duke recovered the disfigured lead slug from the patient and dropped it with a distinctive ping into a metal pan, Shaw advised him never to forget that sound: "'It is the sweetest sound a surgeon will ever hear.'"[35] Duke would school his own students in years ahead to listen for that sound and be thankful for every life saved.

Little did he know that he and his mentor would be listening for that sound in the months ahead on one of the darkest days in the nation's history.

CHAPTER 9
Meeting the President

The alarm clock rang out early on the morning of November 22, 1963. The life of a surgical resident at Dallas's Parkland Hospital was never for those who like to sleep late. Waking as late as five o'clock made it a good morning. There were patient rounds to make, department meetings, new patients, and always, without fail, the unexpected.

Lying in bed beside Red, breathing softly, was Betty. She wouldn't have to get up for another hour. In less than a month they would be celebrating their tenth wedding anniversary. Down the hall was their five-year-old son, Hank. His full name was Cowden Henry Duke, in honor of both his grandfathers. Behind another door were their two daughters. Rebecca was three, and Sara had just turned one a month ago.

November 22 was also Betty's birthday, her thirty-fifth. In fact, Red had bought ballet tickets for that evening. Not his cup of tea, but this was her birthday and he was happy to give her a break from the kids. She had reluctantly given up a teaching career when Hank came along and was dutifully staying at home, raising the family, and tending to the myriad domestic duties that a surgical resident had little time for or interest in. In four years almost to the day, they would have their fourth child, Hallie. Hallie's arrival in 1967 would complete the family of six. But it would also permanently sideline Betty's hopes of recovering her own career.

A quick predawn glimpse at the morning newspaper reminded Red that President Kennedy was going to be in town today. It would be nice to see the president, but that was out of the question, given the demands of the hospital. Years later Red would recall that he hadn't read enough of the full article to know that the governor of Texas, John Connally, would be travelling with the president as well.

This was Red's third year of postgraduate surgical training. Next year he would be the senior resident. That title was a distinction. It meant that he had been singled out for his promise among many with promise. It also served to remind him that he might be making this drive an hour earlier next year—that is, if he made it home from the hospital at all.

The hours of residency training seemed endless. Some wives with small children at home were known to tape a photo of their medical resident to the refrigerator with a note saying "Children, this is your father. If you see this man in our house, don't be afraid." Fortunately Betty hadn't resorted to that extreme—yet.

Making morning rounds with patients, Red already had a reputation as one of the friendliest and most conversational surgical residents a patient could hope to have. You didn't have to be assigned to his care to get a visit. These patients were his people. He had grown up in Ennis and Hillsboro, "just a few miles down the road" by Texas standards. A patient whose television was tuned into a show like *Gunsmoke* or *Bonanza* could expect a chair to be pulled up and the most affable Texan in the state to unfold into it.

On this morning the chairman of surgery, Tom Shires, was away in Galveston at a medical conference.[1] Now that Red was doing a surgical rotation in thoracic surgery with Robert Shaw, knowledge of his immediate boss's whereabouts mattered. Shaw was at a conference just a mile down the road at Woodland Hospital, an affiliate of UT Southwestern specializing in chest diseases. Sometime after lunch he planned to return to Parkland and the medical school. Red knew how to reach him if he needed to.

Something he didn't know was that at 11:50 that morning, President Kennedy and his wife, Jackie, had departed from Love Field for an eleven-mile motorcade through downtown Dallas. Governor John Connally and his wife, Nellie, were in the jump seat directly in front of them. Jackie, dressed in pink, cradled a bouquet of roses. A light mist had been falling in Fort Worth earlier that morning when the presidential delegation had boarded the quick thirty-mile flight to Dallas. But in Dallas the sky was clearing, and the protective top of the midnight blue 1961 Lincoln carrying the presidential party had been removed. What a difference a little rain in Dallas that morning might have made. John F. Kennedy never wanted the protective bubble separating him from the people. The bulletproof side windows were down, too.

Red Duke had no way of knowing any of this. But he did know it was lunchtime and a quiet Friday around the hospital. He joined the hospital chaplain and some faculty friends in the cafeteria at about the same time that the president's motorcade was leaving Love Field.

As Duke was sitting at the back of Parkland's cafeteria grazing on his sandwich, in a time long before cell phones and pagers, the hospital's public address system came to life. It was 12:31 and the urgency of the voice drew his attention. "Calling Dr. Shires, STAT. Dr. Shires's Staff, STAT." Duke knew immediately something was up.

> I was eatin' lunch, which is pretty unusual, with Chaplain Pepper in the Parkland dining room. Just a great big ole dining room, and they started paging Dr. Shires's staff. We didn't have beepers, just overhead paging, and I'd never heard them page the head of surgery that way. I got up and walked over to the phone, and Ron Jones [another surgery resident] got there just before I did. He turned around and said, "Come on. Don't look excited." "Well, hell. I am excited. What's there to be excited about?" I remember motioning to the guys at our table. They were eating. Ron said, "The president's been shot, and I think—I don't know, but I think this is true." I thought to myself, "Well, I'm going to get to meet a president. I never met one of them."
>
> We went out kinda the back door of it, and I was on the thoracic surgery service at the time. We walked past, just walked down the hall a little bit, and there was this little tiny room you'd call an office or the library, and I tried to call Dr. Shaw, who I consider my godfather in all this stuff. There was nobody there. You know, it was lunch, and nobody was in his office. So I went on downstairs and walked through this kinda holding area and x-ray, and I'd never seen so many people in there, and that impressed me, and I walked on into the emergency room. It was totally empty. I'd never seen that. Made a right turn and started as far as from here to that door [a few steps] to go into trauma, and on the right side was where Trauma Room 1 was. I saw Jackie Kennedy sitting beside the door and her pink suit was stained with blood. The seriousness of the event started to sink in. I walked in there, and

there were these three guys—Malcolm Perry, Charlie Baxter, and Robert McClelland—working on the president's throat. Another man was doin' a cut down on his ankle.

Apparently, there were a couple of others in the room and I just automatically put on a pair of gloves and walked around behind the president, in other words, standing at the head of the bed, and he had this great big hole in his head. It just was gone. I have no earthly idea of what I said, but they said, "There's a guy across the hall needs some help." Well, I thought, "Shit, I can't do anything. I can do as much over there as I can here." So I just pulled those gloves off and—you know what a kick basin is? It's a rolling disposal can in the operating room. It was sittin' over there in the corner, and I remember so clearly those cream-colored gloves falling over the inverted stems of Jackie Kennedy's roses, and I remember them bein'—I think they were red. I'm pretty sure they were red. I will never forget the sad sight of my surgical gloves lying on top of those beautiful roses. That was the end of that. I just walked over there and got busy with this fella I soon found out was the governor of Texas.[2]

Duke rolled the governor's gurney into Trauma Room 2, across the hall from the president, who would receive last rites and be pronounced dead at 12:55 p.m. by Dr. Kemp Clark, a neurosurgeon. Connally suffered from bullet wounds to the chest, wrist, and thigh. Whether it was a single bullet or multiple bullets was of little interest at this point compared to saving the governor's life. That question, however, would fuel more than a few conspiracy theories in the years ahead.

Along with fellow resident James Boland, Red placed a tight occlusive dressing on the chest wound, inserted a rubber tube between the second and third ribs in the front right chest to inflate the right lung, drew blood for cross-matching, and notified the operating room on the floor above to get ready as they awaited the arrival of their division chief, Robert Shaw.[3] "Once we got the governor's lung inflated," recalls Red, "he looked around and started talking." Shaw's testimony before the Warren Commission's investigation of that day's events picks up his story as he left Woodland Hospital, returning to Parkland.

As I was driving toward the medical school I came to an
intersection of Harry Hines Boulevard and Industrial Boulevard. There is also a railroad crossing at this particular point.
I saw an open limousine pass this point at high speed with a
police escort. We were held up in traffic because of this escort.
Finally, when we were allowed to proceed, I went on to the
medical school expecting to eat lunch. I had the radio on
because it was the day that I knew the president was in Dallas
and would be eating lunch at the Trade Mart which is not far
away, and over the radio I heard the report that the president
had been shot at while riding in the motorcade. I went on
to the medical school, and as I entered the medical school a
student came in and joined three other students, and said the
president has just been brought into the emergency room at
Parkland, dead on arrival. The students said, "You are kidding
aren't you?" And he said, "No, I am not. I saw him, and Governor Connally has been shot through the chest." Hearing that I
turned and walked over to the emergency room.[4]

In a 1972 interview with Red recalling the governor's surgery nine years
earlier, the *Atlantic Monthly* magazine reported that Shaw "came in on
them, and wanting to know the medical situation, asked Duke, 'Well,
what do we have here?' 'The Governor of Texas,' Duke replied. The governor sat up, stuck out his hand and said, 'John Connally, glad to meet
you.' The doctors had to ease him back down, telling him he was not well
enough to politick."[5]

John Connally survived. Red Duke would not make it home that
night. Betty would be alone with her children. Like the rest of the nation,
Betty and the children huddled in front of the television throughout the
weekend. They also waited to hear from Red.

A secluded room was prepared for Governor and Mrs. Connally, with
Red instructed by Secret Service to stay by the governor's side. Red would
not return home for four days. Meanwhile, he and the Connallys came to
know and like each other. Their friendship would last their lifetimes.

Just six weeks after that terrible day in Dallas, Red received a handwritten note from the Executive Mansion in Austin. It was an expression

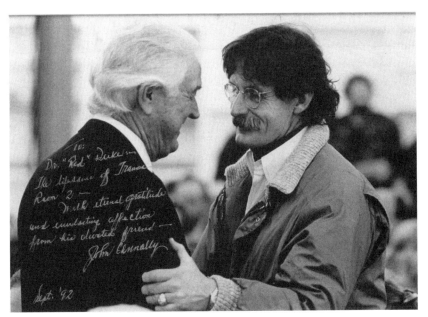

Photo in Red's office signed by John Connally in 1992 in appreciation of Red's lifesaving efforts three decades earlier when President Kennedy and then Governor Connally were rushed to Parkland Hospital.

of appreciation to the man who had saved the governor's life. The note was typical of many exchanges over the years between the Dukes and the Connallys: "Please accept our heartfelt thanks for your kind and thoughtful expressions of friendship, prayer and hope when we both needed them so much. John & Nellie Connally" (January 9, 1963).

Recalls Betty, "My birthday certainly took backstage to the events of that Friday in Dallas. I explained to the children that their father could not come home for a while as he was taking care of a patient. Rebecca was only three at the time, but I'll never forget her little words, 'Something very bad has happened.'" Two days later, on Sunday morning, Betty's brother, George, and sister, Mary Jane, joined her watching news reports and waiting for word from Red. They, like millions of Americans across the nation, watched on live TV as Lee Harvey Oswald walked across their screen and was shot.

Hank was just five. He watched intently as he heard that the president's assassin would be taken to Parkland Hospital where the same doctors would go back to work. Betty was stunned by the words Hank blurted out: "I hope he dies; I want my daddy to come home."[6]

It was half a century before Red talked very much about the events of that day in Dallas. When the fiftieth anniversary of the assassination came around, only a few of the physicians who were there that day were still alive. Then, in media interview after interview, he told his story.

CHAPTER 10

A Texan in New York

Red Duke found strong surgical mentors in Dallas at UT Southwestern. Robert Shaw, the son of a Methodist minister, was one of the best thoracic surgeons around, and he had a medical missionary's commitment to work as much as possible in a part of the world that needed all the help it could get: Afghanistan. In Kabul he had been a teaching surgeon. Shaw was a humanitarian who was sure of his skill and bent on sharing it with sufferers far from the comforts of Dallas. His dedication captured Red's attention, and his experiences stirred the younger surgeon to expand his surgical capabilities.

Shaw told Duke that in Afghanistan he had felt the lack of a stronger background in orthopedics. "That got me interested in orthopedics," Duke said. "In the fourth year of my residency training I did two rotations of orthopedics. When the chairman of orthopedics lost a couple of his residents, he offered to give me the service if I would come back, with the restriction that I could not operate on necks and some hands."[1] But Red turned down the offer to become an orthopedic surgeon in favor of continuing to study general surgery and acquiring a mastery of internal medicine. That combination would carry him through the greatest number of situations he was likely to encounter in any corner of the world.

At the same time, mentors like Tom Shires, the chairman of surgery at UT Southwestern, were encouraging him with their conviction that he would be a great surgeon as well as a great researcher and teacher. In short, Duke said, "They started talking to me about staying on the faculty." Duke concluded that he would in fact do more good in the world by teaching medicine to many people than he would by limiting his contribution to what he could do with his own pair of hands.[2] And when he finished his residency, although he did not give up his dream of becoming a medical missionary, he did join the faculty of UT Southwestern. He started as an instructor in 1965. Within a year he was an assistant professor in pursuit of a research fellowship to widen his areas of expertise. "At that point," he said, "we had no way to feed people that could not eat. They were starving to death. The rudimentary knowledge we had was they just mobilized their body nitrogen. Their urine nitrogen goes way up. It just melts. And so, I got interested in metabolism and that sort of thing and started looking around. My proposal was to get into protein metabolism. One of the real heroes of the day was a guy named Franny Moore at the Brigham."[3]

Francis "Franny" Moore had been on the staff at Massachusetts General on the night of November 28, 1942, when one of the deadliest fires in the country's history broke out in Boston at the Cocoanut Grove nightclub. The fire started around 10:15 that night, by best estimates, and even now the cause is debated.[4] What is known is that the flames moved faster than the patrons. By morning 492 people were dead and hundreds more were severely burned.

Many advancements in burn care were born that night in Boston as hundreds of victims were rushed to Massachusetts General and Boston City Hospitals. At Mass General, Francis Moore was one of the surgeons who innovated with fluid resuscitation techniques for the burn patients. Their treatments with soft gauze covered with petroleum jelly instead of tannic acid proved by far more effective than the more traditional techniques used at Boston City. Advances in blood banking also proved their value that night, as did a new antibiotic now known as penicillin, which demonstrated its ability to combat infections that typically plagued skin grafts at the time.

Francis Moore's experience with the burn victims of the Cocoanut Grove quickened his interest in critical care and the composition of bodily fluids. At the time of the fire, many medical decisions about postoperative care, such as whether a patient needed more fluids, were largely guesswork. It was to eliminate the guesswork that Moore focused his research on chemicals and fluid composition. To determine how levels of water, potassium, sodium, nitrogen, blood, and the like change during surgery, he monitored them with radioactive tracer elements.[5] The results were lifesaving for patients worldwide. Moore's textbook *The Metabolic Care of the Surgical Patient* was published in 1959, just as Red Duke was about to finish medical school.[6] That book would be a well-worn fixture in Duke's office for many years.

When Duke showed up to talk to Moore, however, "he just did not have anything going in the protein area."[7] But a former trainee of his, John M. Kinney (1921–2011), was doing work at Columbia that Moore thought might be just the ticket. And it was.

Moore's influence had inspired Kinney to design a system that would combine the care and study of critically ill patients. In 1963 Kinney had gone to New York–Presbyterian/Columbia University Medical Center, and there he had developed and built the Surgical Metabolism Unit (SMU), a highly successful system that did indeed facilitate both treatment and research. The SMU constituted a new approach to studying the role of nutrition and metabolic care in the recovery of the extremely ill. Equipment in the patient rooms and in the adjacent labs allowed for meticulous measurements of metabolic function and provided an extra layer of monitoring that set patient care apart from the traditional intensive care of the time.

Kinney's timing was ideal for a surgeon like Red, interested in developing an advanced understanding of a rapidly advancing field. In 1966 the National Institutes of Health (NIH) launched a national research program focused on trauma and chose Columbia's SMU as the flagship unit. The associated funding provided postdoctoral training for over forty residents and fellows across the United States and internationally.

Red invoked his chairman Tom Shires's blessing to apply for an NIH grant, which he won. With it he would be able to join John Kinney at Columbia for what he and Shires agreed would probably be one year, during which he could continue his research into protein metabolism. He would at the same time get relevant additional training in mathematical modeling and computer science. Then he would return to Dallas and a long career at Southwestern. Shires arranged for Southwestern to pay him all summer, but the school would make no arduous demands on him for the paychecks.

In the spring of 1967, Red worked out an arrangement to move Betty and the children to New York. He would have no trouble remembering the date of the move; it coincided with the Arab-Israeli Six-Day War, which was commanding international headlines. As a tanker, he told Betty confidently that the war would be brief because the Egyptians would not know how to maintain tanks in the desert sand. "You've got to regrease every bearing every day with fresh grease until it comes out on the other side or it will just wear them out," he said.[8] And he proved right.

There was not much money for the move. Red's salary during his early training in Dallas had been less than a hundred dollars a month, and unlike his family, it had grown little over time.[9] Even now, the Dukes were living paycheck to paycheck, despite help from both sets of parents. There was packing to do, and Betty's mother drove up to Dallas from Pearsall to pitch in and help her pregnant daughter with the work. Red, however, took off to visit an artist friend, Reveau Bassett, who, he vowed, was available to be visited at that moment and no other. Betty and her mother packed the two cars to the hilt with all the belongings that would fit in them. The family went in one car; someone else drove the other to New Jersey, where they met. It was a long, hot, un-air-conditioned drive made with three small children in a tightly packed space. With all of that and her pregnancy, and no doubt some resentment at Red's defection during packing, the trip could not have been a pleasant one for Betty.

Hot as the drive from Texas had been, the very tip of Long Island where Betty and the children settled was cold: "June on Long Island felt like wintertime to us Texans." During that summer Betty was occupied with unpacking, moving in, taking care of the children and the house, and trying to keep warm. "The children would go outside and hunt for limbs and sticks to burn in the fireplace to add heat to the house. Oh, it could get cold out there on the end of Long Island, even in the summer."[10] Red could not be of much help—he was home only on weekends, because when they had arrived in New York, the family had split up for the rushed summer months before them. Red had headed straight for Columbia and the brush-up classes in calculus and computer science that he would need for his work with John Kinney. While Betty and the children shivered on Long Island, Red found it hot in the city:

> That first summer, I lived in the dormitory of the medical students. It was not air-conditioned. I can tell you that New York does get hot in the summertime. My family lived out on the end of Long Island in South Hole for a few months when we first arrived, and I would ride the Long Island Railroad to see them. I took one year of calculus that summer and I had not looked at a math book in you can imagine how many years. I love math but I had to learn to think in those terms again. It

took me a little while to get rolling. It was pretty funny—that first morning I walked in the class at Columbia College, this is right before the 1968 riots—I was still trying to look like a professor, you know. I had a tie on and all that. I was a little out of place. I walked in there, sat down, and this guy, an Israeli mathematician, is teaching. I could not understand anything that guy was saying. I got up, went back downstairs to check to be sure I was in the right room. I was. But I finally got to rolling on it and I just kept going to school taking advanced math and took some engineering courses and I learned to write Fortran. I am a poor computer nut now. Our computer was an old IBM 1100. It was about as long as from here to the door. It sounded like a thrashing machine with all those cards.

In the afternoons I was working in the Department of Biochemistry with Dr. David Rittenberg, who had brought mass spectrometry to America. Ironically, when I was stationed in Meitz, Germany, that town was just a bombed out little

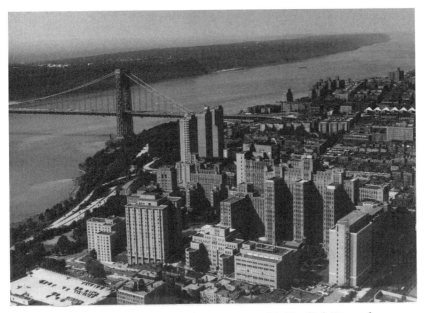

Columbia University and Columbia Presbyterian Hospital in New York City, early 1970s. Photo by Elizabeth Wilcox. Courtesy Archives and Special Collections, Columbia University Health Sciences Library.

nothing. Well, that's the very place mass spectrometry was invented.

So I was setting up this lab and what we were doing was giving N15 [a rare stable isotope of nitrogen] labeled alanine to patients and collecting their urine. I did this by myself. Lord only knows how many samples I went through. We did the urea, the ammonia, and the total nitrogen on all of those samples and with that we were going to develop a mathematical model of amino acid metabolism. They had this Danish engineer, a chemical engineer, and they were the only ones that knew anything about mathematical models in those days. I was enjoying it, you know, having a good time.[11]

In the fall the Dukes found a house in Mount Vernon, just north of the Bronx and closer to the city. Rebecca, eight at the time, remembers it fondly. "That was the house we lived in when Hallie was born. My room was at the top of the stairs. While my mother was in the hospital delivering Hallie, I remember my dad was in charge of making dinner for his three children at home. It seemed kind of silly if not downright funny to us when he served us scrambled eggs. In hindsight, it was probably the only thing he knew how to make back then for children to eat."[12]

But it was not easy to get comfortable and settle in, because by the end of the first year, budget cuts in Congress made funding for Red's grant look wobbly. Red called the NIH, and the response was not reassuring. However, the unsettling alarm turned out to be a false one; the grant was in fact renewed, and Betty broke the good news to Red's parents in Hillsboro: "We got the grant and it is 'full pay.' Red certainly was relieved and has been some relaxed (even though he has his final in calculus on Thursday). The man who talked to him about the grant congratulated him saying the competition was very keen" (August 29, 1968).

The second year would find the Dukes renting a farmhouse at 51 Willow Road, Closter, New Jersey. It belonged to a Columbia faculty member who was taking a sabbatical. The house was situated beautifully on two acres and abutted a wildlife preserve where two ponds nestled. The name Closter is Dutch and comes from the word "Kloos," meaning "a quiet place, a monastery or cloister." Compared to the house out on Long Island, where they had to scavenge for firewood to keep warm, Betty found the Closter farmhouse snug and comfortable. Red was home more now, since he was running a research lab and taking classes rather than being on call night and day for surgery. The Dukes watched sunsets and planted a garden, enjoying the first real family time that they had had in their married life. "It was a wonderful home," Betty said. "I told Red this was just the kind of place I could stay." They planned vacations and took weekend trips together. Betty's mother and an aunt came for a visit, and life seemed very normal.[13] But the halcyon days could not last forever, because Red's career was still unsettled.

During the second year of the grant, Kinney offered Duke an opportunity to stay at Columbia permanently and take over running the entire metabolic clinic. Duke did not want the job, but he thought twice when Kinney dangled the promise of a promotion to associate professor, which he said he could arrange.[14] Duke foresaw that the position would be time-consuming and troublesome ("there are a lot of crazy problems related to this job"), but he felt an obligation to Kinney, who very much needed him to take it—"desperately" needed him to, Duke wrote in a letter to Henry, "and I'm going to have to do it" (June 14, 1969). But Duke also felt a conflicting obligation to Tom Shires at Southwestern, where he had agreed to return when his grant was up. In addition, the much-loved house at Closter had been reclaimed by its owners, whose sabbatical was over. An attempt to buy a different house had foundered over the title.

"It seemed like a pretty good deal, but, I mean, I thought I was doing the right thing. I wrote to the chairman of surgery in Dallas [Tom Shires] and asked what would be his advice."[15] No doubt it was an uncomfortable letter to write. Shires did not respond, and the silence from Dallas spoke volumes. "He was an egomaniac and I guess he thought if I had the audacity to do that, to even consider not coming back to Dallas, he would banish me. . . . So I stayed."[16] Returning to Dallas was apparently no longer an option, and staying at Columbia running a busy clinical research program while juggling the endless need for grants and renewals of grants was increasingly unappealing. Red's new position as lab director was to be short-term by his own choice. Something had to change. His career path in medicine had never seemed so uncertain or so troubling, and to make it all more annoying, the promotion to associate professor never came through.

Red Duke had decisions to make during this summer of 1969, and they would determine his future. For both him and the country it was a summer of turmoil. The assassinations of Martin Luther King and Bobby Kennedy and the ongoing war in Vietnam weighed heavy on the nation as college campuses erupted in protests and draft cards burned. On another note that summer, a concert and art fair were being planned on a dairy farm in upstate New York. The town was Woodstock, and the concert is considered by many a cultural turning point for the nation and the defining of a new generation.[17]

As Red Duke pondered his options for his career and his family, his own turning point occurred in the form of a phone call late one evening. On the other end of the line was a voice that caught him by surprise with a proposition that was even more surprising and would take him a world away from Columbia University.

CHAPTER 11
Afghanistan

The voice of rescue on the other end of that fateful late night phone call belonged to Robert Shaw, the Methodist minister's son who had been Duke's teacher and mentor in Dallas. Shaw had taken the lead as together he and Duke saved John Connally's life at Parkland on that terrible day seven years earlier. Duke had kept an eye on his old professor's undertakings:

> I had been following Shaw's work in Afghanistan and knew they were getting a new medical school started in Jalalabad. Now that's a place nobody had heard of until after 9/11. But Robert Shaw knew it well. I asked, "What is going on in Jalalabad?" He said, "That is interesting. We just put a team together to work in that school. It is just getting started. It is just rolling and I volunteered you." I said, "Well, let me tell you, if I can get rid of this house I put money down on, you've got a deal."[1]

Robert Shaw's trips to Afghanistan went back to his days as a medical student, when he had set out on an adventure to see the world. He took with him nothing more than a backpack and a camera and a passion to see and learn everything he could. It was January 1929 when he reached the border of Afghanistan. Later he would tell Dallas reporter James Dunlap that Afghanistan "was closed then and all I was allowed to do was snap a few pictures, but I was so impressed by the rugged country and the rugged people with their guns slung over their shoulders that from then on I went through medical school hoping I could go back sometime."[2]

Shaw left his private practice in Dallas in 1961, at the age of fifty-five, to devote more time to Afghanistan. He had already made many trips there—some short, at least one lasting two years—in the thirty-two years that had elapsed since he had first fallen in love with the country. Now, as a surgeon for MEDICO, "he performed surgery, taught native doctors and medical students, and acted as chief of staff at a new hospital in Kabul. He performed the first heart operation in Afghanistan. His wife, a former nurse, helped set up the hospital's central supply and worked in the recovery room."[3] Busy as he was, Shaw had also found time to start "a forty-bed hospital for medical and surgical chest diseases in Kabul and worked in the country's second medical school, in Jalalabad," where Red would join him for the mission trip in 1970.[4]

The stories Robert Shaw had brought back to UT Southwestern from his trip in 1961 had transfixed Red Duke and idealistic students like him who dreamed of a life in medical service—a life that would exact their personal sweat and sacrifice to relieve suffering among distant people in underdeveloped countries and with unfamiliar cultures. Red's first humanitarian hero had been Schweitzer, whose sacrifices could never be equaled—he had sacrificed half a lifetime of civilization at its pitch. But his immediate hero was Shaw, who would go to Afghanistan eleven times for periods ranging from two weeks to two years. Actually, this trip with Red in 1970 was near the end of Shaw's expeditions. By 1974, when he went for the last time, there was talk of a Russian invasion. It did not materialize until four years later, but already the country was too dangerous. On the 1974 trip, Shaw would have to consult with his former auto mechanic to find out which of his friends he could visit without endangering them.[5]

The 1970 mission trip Robert Shaw asked Red Duke to join had been organized through an agreement between Loma Linda University and the University of Indiana. In 1962 Gordon Hadley, a physician from Loma Linda, had been on assignment in Vellore, India, for the World Health Organization, which asked him to investigate a request from Afghanistan to strengthen the medical schools in Jalalabad and Kabul. From that investigation, a plan emerged in the late 1960s to organize this mission.[6] The team that composed it consisted of seven physicians, along with nurses, support personnel, and a teacher for the children of team members. Once assembled, the team was both eclectic and international, with members from the United States, New Zealand, India, and the Philippines. It was also ecumenical, with four Catholic sisters, several Methodists, a Southern Baptist (Red Duke), one person of Jewish faith, and several Seventh Day Adventists, including the team's leader, Gordon Hadley.

Sister Jane Fell, one of the first members to arrive in Kabul, found that "the team itself was a big source of the joy of being in Afghanistan. We sisters shared fully with those of other faiths, joining their worship services and inviting them to join us for Mass at times. Afghan law forbid proselytizing so Dr. Hadley said we would only declare our Christian faith by our action, that is, by the way we cared for anyone in need. During our stay there we never split over religion. As long as we kept to the deeper levels of all of our faiths, we were united."[7]

This arrangement suited Duke very well. He considered a medical missionary's mission to be medical, not evangelistic. He respected his patients' culture and had no interest in attempting to change their religion. Hallie remembers that years later, when she was an adult with children of her own, he lectured her on the distinction between missionary programs that are faith-oriented and those that are service-oriented. Press releases also emphasized that the team would not proselytize. Its goal was better medical care for people in need.[8]

Duke had accepted the position from Shaw after talking it out with Betty, who was in favor of it, too. Undertaking a foreign mission had been after all a great dream of theirs as young lovers, and Betty saw Afghanistan as the fulfillment of that dream. But the difficult realities of life in Afghanistan, particularly with children in tow, were going to set in on her within a few months, and she would lay out a strong case for staying only one year. Duke, however, would argue that their purpose could not be fulfilled in less than two years, and he would prevail, leaving Betty with a sense that she had been overruled and was no longer an equal partner in the relationship. Reluctantly she put another year's hold on her dreams of a perfect family life.

With some difficulty the Dukes divested themselves of the house in New Jersey that they had paid down on. They enlisted a young school teacher, Chloe Stacey, whom Betty knew from Pearsall, Texas, to go along as tutor for the children. And they persuaded Red's administrative assistant at Columbia, Jill Hoffman, to join the venture as administrative support. In the fall of 1970, Red Duke and family set foot on Afghan soil. Betty must have felt like Neil Armstrong setting foot on the moon (which he had done just months before). In any case, this was the service opportunity they had dreamed of, and it was also a chance to expose the children to a new culture and a very different world. Hank was now twelve; Rebecca, ten; Sara, eight; and Hallie, two.

For the next two years Betty would run the house and manage the children, and Duke would shuttle the eighty miles between Kabul and their home base in Jalalabad, performing surgery and teaching. In Kabul they met new friends and stocked up on household supplies. An American internist, Austin Moede, and his family were in Kabul at the time, and the two families became close. From his home in Albuquerque more than four decades later, Moede (pronounced Meady) recalls wonderful times with the Dukes. When in need of medical care himself or a second opinion, Red would often turn to Moede, who recalls an injury Red sustained playing flag football. He "had torn up his knee one day and showed up in Kabul limping with a large contusion." With children running around in Moede's garden and wives chattering with one another to catch up on events in this small world, Red submitted his knee to a thorough evaluation by a "committee" of physician friends and pronounced it fit to recover on its own if Red would just slow down. Recalls Moede soberly, "I said amongst all of us we could do just about anything known to medicine with his knee, but the one thing I would not do was drain it with a needle. The risk of introducing an infection through an unnecessary procedure was just not worth it and something always to be considered with a patient in Afghanistan."[9]

When he was not seeing patients, Red lectured in Afghanistan more than he ever had. In addition to performing those traditional duties, he dealt with the medical equipment, which was archaic and rickety. He spent time "trying to jerry-rig stuff, you know, because it was pretty primitive."[10] He found himself doing what he had practiced in Boy Scouts and as a tank commander—namely, making creative use of whatever was at hand to fill in for what was missing. If he had to find a pulley and cord to create a makeshift contraption to raise a patient's arm or leg, he did it. This did not annoy him; in fact, he enjoyed practicing his ingenuity. Nevertheless, amid all the work, Red was becoming increasingly aware of how small the team really was for the size of the task at hand. After the first year, Dr. Shaw was gone. That left five physicians besides Red. Of these, two were interns, one was a bacteriologist who worked in the lab, one a pathologist, and one a Fulbright scholar who taught physiology.

The two years in Afghanistan were brutal, challenging, exciting, rewarding, and eye-opening for Duke. He was on his feet day and night.

Betty worried constantly that he needed more rest. Duke described his days in a letter home:

> We are working very hard at the hospital. . . . The surgery problems are abundant. I am really doing general surgery. I am doing quite a lot of urology, orthopedics, and plastics as well as general surgery. I had no idea I could be so busy. . . .

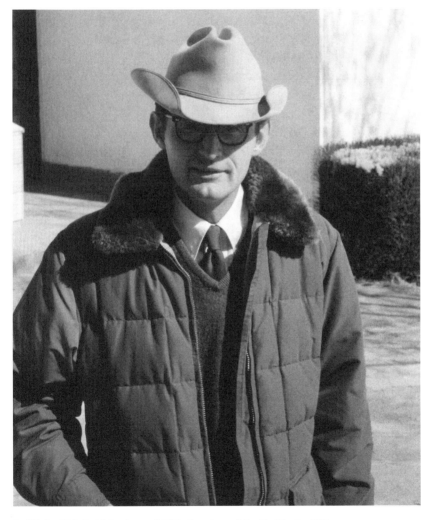

Red Duke, Kabul, Afghanistan, 1971. Courtesy of Austin Moede, MD.

I had to do an internal fixation of a fractured femur this
morning. I just finished my usual late lunch of nan, the local
Afghan bread, cheese, and tea. I have never been where I
could have lunch at home. I am far busier than I had expected
and therefore do not have as much time at home as I would
like. (December 29, 1971)

Sister Jane Fell was an outgoing Iowa farm girl who had completed her
nursing degree in Omaha and had taken her vows as a nun through
the Society of Medical Mission Sisters. She was the first member of
the team to reach Afghanistan in 1970. Her memoirs, self-published
in 2011, give a first-hand glimpse of life in Afghanistan as the team
and their families experienced it. Red Duke won her admiration early
on: "We were blessed," she writes, "by having excellent surgeons on the
team. . . . Dr. Duke was both an orthopedic and vascular surgeon. He
was able to reconstruct and save limbs . . . that in my past experience
were usually amputated."[11] Medical students were learning not only in
the classroom but also by attending these surgeries, which they participated in. "The university hospital," Sister Fell wrote, "soon became a
place to which patients from other parts of the country could be referred
for specialty care."[12]

Betty stayed busy with her domestic duties and took classes in Farci.
At first she was overcome by the "dust and dirt. . . . Everything appeared
dirty and poor: the people, the animals, the houses, and especially the
roads." But once she grew used to that, she reported in an open letter
to friends and family that she found "beautiful people under the many
dusty clothes. We are getting used to the unpaved, bumpy streets; and
in fact we are beginning to feel very much 'at home,' though we still
do not understand anyone yet." She adds, "Two neighborhood ladies
came to visit me one morning. They spoke in Farsi (Persian); I spoke in
English; we both smiled a lot; I patted the children; and they left. Now
we always wave to each other, and I hope we are friends" (November 28,
1970).

The house, although it was new—in fact, it was still being finished out when they moved in—had its eccentricities. It was "built of
and surrounded by a wall of concrete (to use the term loosely)" and it
crumbled on impact with objects like furniture. The hot running water

was confined to the bathroom, the landlord having expressed his opinion that putting it in the kitchen too would be redundant, so that to have hot water in the kitchen, someone had to carry it from the bath or heat it on the stove. Betty was grateful to have it anywhere. There were certain decorative issues as well. "The floors downstairs," she wrote, "are made of tile—and on our living room floor there are three different patterns—just not enough of one to do the entire floor, we suppose. The walls were painted with rags, using a whitewash type of paint that comes off on our clothes. So much for our 'falling-apart, new house.' Dr. Shaw says that Afghanistan is the only country he knows of that builds ruins!"

The food, however, was another matter:

> We eat very well here—maybe even better than we did at
> home, certainly not as expensively nor as easily. We get lots
> of fruit and vegetables and some meat, which is not too good.
> The English walnut originated in Afghanistan; almonds are
> also plentiful. Because most of the food has been dipped in
> contaminated water, we wash everything in soap and water,
> then soak it in an iodine solution for twenty minutes. Then it
> is ready to eat raw or cooked. Our cook has worked for Ameri-
> cans before and knows how to prepare all the food and how to
> keep the water boiled for drinking. He also is very compulsive
> about keeping the house swept and mopped.

"He's great!!" she concluded, with more enthusiasm than accuracy, as it would turn out. Soon after sending the letter she developed typhoid fever and was ill for weeks. "I finally figured out what he was doing. He was squeezing oranges and washing the sieve in unsafe tap water. When I questioned him about it he said, 'I only let a little water through the strainer.'"[13]

There was no separate church building; services were held in team members' homes. The medical school was off on Fridays, Friday being the Muslim day of worship, so it became the team members' day, too. Similarly, school was held at school teacher Chloe Stacey's house. There were seven students, all but two of them in different grades, but Stacey was up to juggling their lessons accordingly. With help around the house and the children off at school, Betty hoped things would settle down enough that she and Red could spend more time together. But his hospital labors were "grueling," she reported. "I had hoped that life would move more slowly for us here, but not so for the doctor" (November 28, 1970).

Nevertheless, Betty had no trouble filling her time. The Duke house was always full of people. Duke convinced his parents to come for a visit, and his letters were crowded with travel tips, suggestions for packing, guidelines for vaccinations, and advice for sleeping on the plane in order to be rested upon arrival. Betty was able to get her mother and aunt to come, too. Between family visits, the Duke household was a constant hub for other visitors as well, and Betty took on all the duties of hosting guests. Often the visitors were total strangers, mostly young people traveling through in search of a hot meal and a bath. The Duke family home was always open.[14]

In summer, Jalalabad, at an elevation of 1,886 feet, was much hotter than Kabul, which was just shy of 6,000 feet. Much of the university shut down in Jalalabad to move up to Kabul's cooler temperatures. Usually the vacant home of a team member or Peace Corps volunteer could be arranged in Kabul as a place for the family to escape the heat, meet with friends, and stock up on supplies. Betty was more than ready.

On the way between the towns, there was a cooling-off place. "The locals knew a spot on the Khyber River [where] they could pull the car off and climb down a steep cliff to jump in the river to cool down. I'm talking clothes and all, then scale the cliff back to the car. One day it was so hot I suggested to Red we do the same. It was wonderful. I'll never forget how hot it could get over there."[15]

Home schooling for the children moved from Jalalabad to Kabul without issue for the most part. Of course, like all children, the young Dukes found play more appealing than study. But in the end Betty would look back with satisfaction on the fact that that when her children returned to the states, they were all on grade level with their stateside peers.

In a letter to her parents at the end of the first summer, as the family was preparing to move back to Jalalabad from the respite of Kabul, Betty wrote:

Because we have not yet returned to Jalalabad, I am helping
the children with their school work. I feel like we have a four-
ring circus going on all of the time. It really is terribly frustrating to me and to the children. It is hard for them to con-
centrate with all the interruptions we have around here. . . .
I'll be glad to be settled soon. (In fact it's hard for me to write
a decent letter because I'm going from one child to the other
and answering the phone and door in between." (August 15,
1971)

One letter home from Red to his parents just four months after their
arrival in Afghanistan followed up on Betty's constant concern that
he needed more rest. Betty was troubled, and not without reason. Her
husband's usually abundant energy had deserted him. Tasks that had
previously seemed trivial had become major undertakings. She was
recovering from her bout with typhoid fever—no easy task on any continent. Now something was wrong with Red. Eventually he diagnosed
the problem himself and confided it in his parents:

It finally began to dawn on me what was wrong and my internist friend concurred. I had hepatitis. For several days I was
not too chipper. I finally became mildly jaundiced and this has
now begun to recede. I feel very well now but I am easily tired.
I have more respect for the disease than you can imagine and
I will be very faithful about my convalescence. I do not know
how I got it. I had a big dose of gamma globulin before we left,
but I was about due another. The kids and Betty have now had
their second dose. I will assure you I will be careful. (March
10, 1971)

In time Red recovered, but not without bed rest and being knocked out
of action for a month. Another physician friend in Kabul was a special-
ist in treating hepatitis, but getting to Kabul from Jalalabad during Red's
recovery was not easy. Forty treacherous miles of the eighty-mile drive
go through the Kabul Gorge, also referred to by the locals as "the Valley of Death." In 2010, Dexter Filkins, writing for the *New York Times*,
described it:

The 40-mile stretch, a breathtaking chasm of mountains and cliffs between Kabul and Jalalabad, claims so many lives so regularly that most people stopped counting long ago. Cars flip and flatten. Trucks soar to the valley floor. Buses play chicken; buses collide.

The mayhem unfolds on one of the most bewitching stretches of scenery on all the earth. The gorge, in some places no more than a few hundred yards wide, is framed by vertical rock cliffs that soar more than 2,000 feet above the Kabul River below. Most people die, and most cars crash, while zooming around one of the impossible turns that offer impossible views of the crevasses and buttes.[16]

Driving one of the most dangerous highways in the world to get Duke to Kabul during the hepatitis episode forged a memory that decades on still makes Betty's heart drop.

In addition to personal issues like typhoid and hepatitis, a number of things also went awry in the medical community in the course of the mission, ranging from the trivial to the frightening. A baby-weighing program backfired. The team members were weighing babies to identify the underweight ones, for whom they were giving out extra food. They soon discovered that some enterprising pilferers were "borrowing" underweight babies, having them weighed, and making off with the free food.[17]

A more serious problem arose from the inequality of salaries paid to American and Afghan doctors and nurses. Afghan doctors made twenty or thirty dollars a month and were obliged to augment their income by practicing outside the hospital and by taking payment from their hospital patients. "We team members came along," Sister Fell wrote, "giving care free of charge and at all hours of the day or night because we didn't need to make money off the patients. This set us up to experience a lot of jealousy."[18] For this and whatever other reasons, the animosity between Afghan and team staff grew steadily worse. One of the most alarming clashes, Sister Fell reported, arose over a tape recorder:

Our doctors were supposed to have some control over the medical school. Staff meetings were supposed to be in English, a language spoken well by all the professors. But when things became difficult, the Afghan doctors would switch to Farsi/ Persian, and talk fast enough that even our doctors who knew something of the language couldn't follow. So one day our youngest doctor carried a tape recorder with him, and when they switched languages, he put it on top of the desk and turned it on, thinking that he could translate what was being discussed later. After a few minutes the tape recorder was noticed, and the place exploded. They screamed at him that he had done a terrible thing that deserved grave punishment. He removed the tape and tried to give it to them, but they acted as if it was a bomb.[19]

Duke was in the meeting. Of all the faculty meetings he attended in his life, none could ever match the fury unleashed on that day. "The faculty," he wrote home, "deteriorated immediately into a wild, screaming tirade and they were up, running around in and out of the room, screaming, and about all that was recorded was this war dance. When the Dean told [the young faculty member] to turn [the recorder] off, he did and gave the tape to him, but it was impossible to do anything after that and so we left again, only to find that one of these men had slashed and ruined one tire each on some of our cars" (September 29, 1971).

After a year in Afghanistan, Duke was made chair of the medical school's surgical department by the president and the senior administration of Nangarhar University (in Jalalabad, where most of his work was centered). Many of the Afghan physicians bitterly resented an American's having authority over them, and they raised vigorous objections to Duke's appointment. In a letter home, Duke wrote that "Hadley [the mission team leader] objected to the president of the university that this group had no business discussing this issue and it was a violation of our contract with the government, and the president agreed that it should not be discussed except with the administration." Nevertheless, discuss it they did. They based their displeasure on Duke's qualifications, although his training and surgical experience far exceeded those of even the most senior of the Afghan surgeons. Faculty meetings became long and confrontational. At one of them, when the ostensible intent was to address Duke's qualifications, he thought the real intent was "to make life tough on me and embarrass the team."

One of the most difficult and trying issues of the day was student grades. Red saw that unqualified students were being advanced, even graduated, and he would have none of it. The environment was such that he doubted the renewal of his contract, but he would not relent. He shared his frustration with his parents: "My position is still somewhat confused because I am unwilling to accept a compromise made concerning the passing of a bunch of ineligible students in surgery. Only time can resolve this problem. I did not know that we could get into so much trouble with so little effort. I hope when I leave here, whenever that occurs, they will at least know that one hard head did not believe in permitting dishonest acts to go unnoticed" (November 3, 1971). Weeks later he was still battling: "You cannot believe the number of hours we have wasted fighting these terribly short-sighted, spineless faculty members trying to make them do the honest straight-forward things. I am afraid it is useless. . . . It is going to be a tough fight in the next few weeks. I would not be surprised if they run us off. Keep a candle in the window" (December 1, 1971).

Red had been in the fight more than a few months. Two months earlier in a letter home, he had reported that he had actually submitted a formal letter "temporarily withdrawing" from the university until "several issues [could] be satisfied" related to student grading. At that time, four students the faculty had failed showed up for an exam he was administering, for which they were ineligible. "The Dean and Vice Dean and two Afghans were illegally present in the hall as proctors. I got the eligible students seated and started but finally these four dissidents created enough furor with the Dean that the Vice Dean finally told the students it was an illegal examination and they all left." Red was told later he did not understand the rules, "i.e., that the Dean can change any chief of department's grade and that this silly faculty can change anything the Dean does" (September 29, 1971). Red clearly was not going to win in such a system, and he turned his greater attention from the classroom to the operating room, where patients needed and wanted his help. Here his qualifications spoke loud and clear.

• • •

In July 1972, John and Nellie Connally showed up in Afghanistan. By this time Connally was secretary of the treasury under Richard Nixon.

James P. Sterba reported for the *New York Times* on the Connallys' reunion with Duke:

> "Red" Duke . . . came to Afghanistan two years ago to help set up a medical faculty at Nangarhar University in Jalalabad, east of Kabul. The Connallys lost track of him for several years, but learned he was in Afghanistan and insisted he be in Kabul when they arrived here on their 17-nation tour for President Nixon.
>
> It was a warm reunion. Mrs. Connally gave Dr. Duke a big hug and Mr. Connally, coming out of a meeting with government officials, said to them: "With all due respect, he is the most important man around here—he saved my life."
>
> Between a luncheon with the King, Mohammad Zahir Shah, and official meetings Mr. Connally and Dr. Duke visited three gun shops. Kabul is famous for its antique and fake antique guns and both men are enthusiastic hunters and collectors.
>
> At a second shop [Connally] said, "Red, have you ever seen such a collection of guns as this before?" Dr. Duke replied: "In the tribal areas like where I live there's even more. Everybody carries them and they're all loaded. I spend a good bit of time taking care of the results."[20]

When his two years were up, Red Duke was ready. Except for the bitter faculty fights, he had loved Afghanistan—its exoticism, its beauty, the beauty of its people. He had seen firsthand medical conditions (leprosy, for instance) that he would rarely have seen at home. He had tested his endurance by working around the clock until he dropped with exhaustion. And he had learned something important about himself, or at least come to suspect it—namely, that he was not and would never be an Albert Schweitzer or even a Robert Shaw. He was willing to work hard and give much. But Schweitzer's love had been for self-sacrifice; Shaw's was for Afghanistan. Duke's was for medicine. He did not want distractions from it. He just wanted to practice medicine. Wherever he practiced it, people were going to benefit from it, and he was going to have succeeded in his ambition to make the world better.

He was ready to go home.

The question was, where was home?

CHAPTER 12

Home to Texas

In the mid-1960s, as Red Duke was joining the faculty of UT South-western after completing his residency, Charles LeMaistre (1924–2017) was already an established faculty member there, in the Department of Internal Medicine. One fall morning in 1965 LeMaistre was surprised to be called from his research lab to the dean's office to meet Harry H. Ransom, the chancellor of the UT System. Ransom had an assignment for LeMaistre that would change the face of Texas health care and the state's capacity for training additional physicians.[1] The results of LeMaistre's work would create a new University of Texas medical school in Houston's Texas Medical Center—a medical school that would provide a new home for Red Duke a few years down the road, when he returned from Afghanistan. LeMaistre recalls:

> The Texas Higher Education Coordinating Board had requested the University of Texas System to undertake a study of the medical needs of this state, projecting to the year 1990. The request was to look at manpower and research activities and to identify how all the medical units of the University of Texas could be enhanced. Thus, the Coordinating Board's request to Harry Ransom resulted in his arrival in Dallas in 1965 to see me. I was a very happy professor of internal medicine, heading a chest disease unit and just enjoying life with very little administrative responsibility.[2]

LeMaistre's report not only identified a need and created a new University of Texas Medical School in Houston; it propelled his career forward in ways he never expected. The University of Texas System would name him vice chancellor of health affairs (1966–69), chancellor (1971–78), and president of the University of Texas M. D. Anderson Cancer Center

(1978–96) following the retirement of the cancer center's founder and visionary leader, R. Lee Clark.

As chancellor, LeMaistre oversaw a university system undergoing rapid growth and on a trajectory to make it one of the leading institutions of higher education in the nation. That rapid growth was in large part due to legislation signed on December 16, 1963, by President Lyndon Johnson, less than a month after that day in Dallas when Johnson ascended to the presidency. Johnson's Higher Education Facilities Act included, among many features, a provision of federal matching funds for construction at public colleges and universities.[3] This mechanism proved essential to the rapid growth of the UT System, including the new medical school planned for Houston's Texas Medical Center.

In 1963 John Connally, then governor of Texas, appointed Frank Erwin (1920–80) to the UT System Board of Regents just days before leaving Austin to join President Kennedy in Dallas. By 1966 Erwin would be chairman and holding the reins of the university's future. Working closely with the state legislature, Erwin increased university appropriations from $40.4 million in 1963/1964 to $349.7 million in 1975/1976.[4]

Erwin was a bulldog of a personality who never took no for an answer and found LBJ's new legislation providing matching funds for

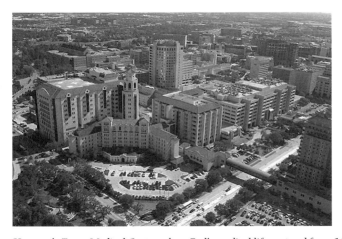

Houston's Texas Medical Center where Red's medical life centered from 1972 until his death in 2015. The red-roofed Hermann Hospital and Life Flight heliport are in the foreground, with connecting McGovern Medical School to the right of the hospital.

building university infrastructure just what he needed. Funds available to any state not able or willing to match designated federal funds could be picked up by other states having the means to match. Thanks to the Permanent University Fund that provided revenues from state-owned, oil-rich land designated to assist both the University of Texas and Texas A&M, Erwin had the means to match and wasted no time in doing so.[5]

A 1948 graduate of the University of Texas School of Law, Erwin took a personal interest not only in building the University of Texas main campus in Austin, but also in building and enhancing the many academic and health components of the UT System throughout the state. High on Erwin's list of priorities in the mid-1960s was the new medical school in Houston, where he wasted no time getting involved in every detail, including the school's affiliation agreement with Hermann Hospital.

As chairman of the UT Board of Regents, Erwin was a powerful man with no shortage of connections and ability. Working from his office in the Ashbel Smith Building in Austin, he planned the new Houston school and, in December 1969, hired its founding dean, Cheves McCord Smythe. Smythe, a Harvard-educated physician from Charleston, South Carolina, arrived with his family in the spring of 1970 to build a new medical school from the ground up.

• • •

On the morning of June 19, 1969, Texas governor Preston Smith came to Houston's Texas Medical Center and signed House Bill 80. With the stroke of the governor's pen, the University of Texas Medical School at Houston was born. Hours later, the governor was in Lubbock, Texas, signing similar documents to create Texas Tech University's new medical school.

At that time Red Duke was in New York at Columbia University, negotiating with his surgical mentor, Robert Shaw, about the opportunity to take his family to Afghanistan.

The governor of Texas may have created a medical school on paper, but it was up to Cheves Smythe to build it, recruit faculty, find students, and establish relationships with affiliate hospitals and medical institutions throughout Houston. This was no small task, but Cheves Smythe was a man who, like Frank Erwin, got things done.

To begin with, Smythe found the building plans entirely inadequate. "I took one look at these plans and was horrified. To me they were obsolete. . . . Large teaching laboratories, an ample library when there was a good one across the street, a book-binding facility, little or no provision for computers, no adequate audiovisual support, lack of a modular design, assumptions about the presence of labs, but above all else no 'program' or conscientious attempt to think through what would be done in the building and to relate that to the plans."[6]

Smythe called for a meeting in Austin with the architects, and Frank Erwin was front and center to offer these encouraging words: "Doctor, you are just like every other damn professor. You think that if you didn't have a hand in the plans, they are no good and have to be changed." Undaunted, even in the face of Frank Erwin, Smythe detailed his concerns and itemized the solutions, to which Erwin replied, "Will you join me in a Coke?"[7]

Remembers Smythe, "I was mystified, but the more experienced people in the room broke out into broad smiles. They knew this was Erwin's signal of approval, and we were given the green light to develop a new set of plans."[8]

Buildings aside, Smythe simultaneously faced the challenge of finding the right leaders for his basic science and clinical departments. Given the many surgical talents already dominating Houston's Texas Medical Center in 1970, Smythe thought carefully about his decisions. His prior deanship at the Medical College of South Carolina, along with his administrative experience as associate director of the Association of American Medical Colleges (AAMC), provided him unique insights regarding the qualities that separated good medical schools from great ones. Recalls Smythe of his search for a surgery chair:

> There were some constraints. M. D. Anderson had cancer surgery pretty well staked out, and locally DeBakey [Michael DeBakey at Baylor College of Medicine across the street] and Denton Cooley [Texas Heart Institute a block farther] were dominant in vascular surgery. I was attracted to Francis Moore's ideas. The department should be built around the theme of the metabolic response to trauma with all surgery defined as trauma.

> At the AAMC I had met and interacted with Jonathan
> Rhoads and had come to admire him literally as much as
> any man I have known. Jonathan was professor of surgery
> at the University of Pennsylvania, main line Philadelphia the
> whole way, a towering figure in American surgery, and on
> every board, committee, and commission. He was a deliberate,
> careful, thoughtful gentleman. I asked his advice about the
> various men we were considering. I say his response was that
> he instructed, not advised me, that we had to choose Stanley
> Dudrick, one of the men he had trained. . . . Jonathan's advice
> was followed and Stan accepted.[9]

In this way, Stanley Dudrick and his family came to Houston to join the new UT medical school. Dudrick had been encouraged by his mentor, Jonathan Rhoads, to solve the problems of malnourished patients, and he had succeeded. Dudrick's successful hyperalimentation technique had made him a star and was saving lives worldwide.

Smythe would find in the early years of the school that Dudrick was just what he needed. "He was a very skillful surgeon. He was positively gifted in the way he dealt with and talked to patients and their families. He had boundless energy, but episodically so, and considerable personal charm. He was a strong leader and attracted and retained good people," Smythe recalled in his memoirs.[10]

Chairmen of the clinical departments at the medical school would also serve as chief of services at Hermann, the school's primary affiliated hospital next door. Smythe's opinion that his new chairman of surgery attracted and retained good people is attested to by Dudrick's early recruits. As Smythe built the school, Dudrick searched for the right people to build his department, and he had some in mind. For starters, he brought along one of the surgical residents who had worked with him on hyperalimentation for the past two years, Bruce MacFadyen Jr. MacFadyen joined the new department as a fourth-year surgical resident and made significant contributions to it for three decades. One of them was his expertise in the emerging field of laparoscopic surgery. He stayed until he was named chairman of surgery in 2002 at Georgia Regents University in Augusta.[11]

Dudrick's eye had been on Ted Copeland since their residency together at the University of Pennsylvania. Copeland was a decorated military surgeon, trained at Duke and Cornell Universities, who had returned from Vietnam to join M. D. Anderson Cancer Center as a fellow in surgical oncology. Copeland's uncle, Murray Copeland, was not only a surgeon and a national leader in the field of colon and large bowel cancer; he was also determined that his nephew not stray too far from the cancer hospital. Ted Copeland joined Dudrick at the new medical school and retained strong ties with the cancer center down the street. A few years later he would return full-time to the cancer hospital, where he had pioneered the use of Dudrick's hyperalimentation techniques for cancer patients and continued his uncle's work as project director for the National Cancer Institute's National Large Bowel Cancer Project. In 1990, he would leave Houston to join the University of Florida's medical school in Gainesville, where he would also serve in other senior administrative capacities.

Also on Dudrick's radar was that young redhead at UT Southwestern who shared an interest in metabolic interventions. Dudrick had not forgotten the young man he had first seen seven years earlier standing in the back of a Dallas lecture hall, focused on every word of Dudrick's talk. Dudrick had been following Duke's career, even hosting him at his house in Philadelphia several times, to learn about the work Duke was doing at Columbia with John Kinney.

Dudrick was impressed with everything he learned about Red Duke, and his letter inviting Red to join the new enterprise in Houston found its way to Jalalabad, where it was received with great interest. Red was tiring of his ongoing battles with the Afghan medical faculty. The long faculty meetings with endless bickering and rows had taken their toll. Additionally, Betty was anxious to get the children back to the States, and now it was plain that Stanley Dudrick wanted Red Duke in Houston—the sooner, the better.

• • •

Red flew to the States for an initial interview and look-around; Betty stayed in Afghanistan with the children. After several days on airplanes en route from Afghanistan, Red was ragged and none too clean when Dean Smythe picked him up at the airport for the first interviews. But all parties liked what they saw. With rented and borrowed space, including lecture halls in the dilapidated Center Pavilion Hospital (no longer in existence), and with an early electron microscope housed in a trailer adjacent to M. D. Anderson's Lutheran Pavilion, Red found the new enterprise just the kind of ground-floor opportunity that appealed to him. In his words, "This was organized chaos, make-it-happen medical education."

Moreover, there was much to admire in this new dean who had taken on the challenge of building a medical school from scratch. Already Smythe had recruited twenty-two medical students and farmed them out to other University of Texas medical schools in Galveston and Dallas. He had promised them buildings and a faculty when they returned for their clinical training in their third year. (In the early days of the school, it was a three-year program.[12])

But Red went to Seattle, Miami, and Denver to look at jobs there, too, before accepting the Houston offer. "They were really recruiting me from Washington and I really loved their program. To this day I do not know why I did not go." Actually, he did know why. "Well, why I came here was because I thought that Stan, Ted, and I were going to continue this really in-depth metabolic stuff. I wanted to build a better metabolic unit than they had in New York, and I enjoyed the research. That was my real intention."[13]

In addition to recruiting early faculty and the first class of twenty-two, Smythe and his new associate dean, Robert Tuttle, addressed the construction of the two-story, 55,000-square-foot John Freeman Building. Just two months after Red had joined the new faculty, President George H. W. Bush, then US ambassador to the United Nations, dedicated the Freeman Building on October 28, 1972, at Houston's Astro-World Hotel. Red and the few dozen faculty now onboard welcomed the new facility, among other reasons because faculty members were each given an academic office and research space. Before the Freeman Building, their offices had resembled closets and were, in addition, in the Texas Medical Center library—which is to say, next door. "Funny to look back," Red said "and remember that we all thought [the Freeman Building] was just the largest building the school would ever need. Even each student had a designated study area." That would change quickly as the school grew and class size increased in the immediate years ahead.

The two-story Freeman Building was actually only a stop-gap

solution. As it was opening, plans were being finalized for a seven-story, 852,000-square-foot medical school building that connected to Hermann Hospital on every floor. Watching the mammoth construction project rise from the ground, Red and the school's early faculty saw the building that had once offered ample accommodation now lost in the shadow of the new building, like a playhouse next to the real thing. In 1976 Red and the department of surgery moved into newer offices on the fourth floor of the completed medical school. Red would fill his space floor-to-ceiling with memorabilia. He would hang deer and bighorn sheep heads on the wall, along with other hunting trophies, and would haul in teaching materials, slide trays, Willie Nelson tapes, beloved textbooks, and patient mementos.

Mixed among these things would be a growing number of awards, especially teaching awards voted by the students, who found Red's commonsense approach to learning refreshing and highly entertaining, as well as to the point. His drawled stories drew on all his experience, from driving tanks through Germany to teaching English to lumberjacks and driving through the Kabul Gorge in Afghanistan, and these tales packed points in such a way that students remembered them. His skills in the operating theater were as impressive as his lectures in the lecture hall,

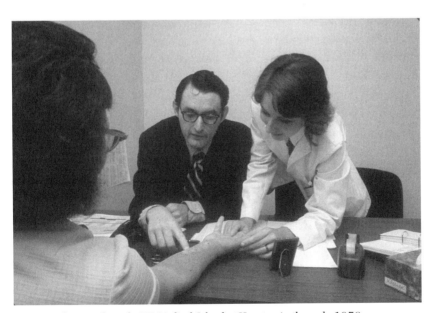

Red in teaching mode at the UT Medical School at Houston in the early 1970s.

according to the students who voted him outstanding teacher over the years.

As the school grew from a three-to a four-year curriculum in September 1977, class size grew. The first class had come back, and nineteen graduated. New classes, bigger every year, followed. In 1977 the school welcomed 150 new medical students, and they would all come to know Red Duke. When he wasn't teaching in the classroom, he was teaching in surgery. A universal sentiment among his students was that you were entertained, you learned, and you wanted to hear more anytime Red Duke was in the room.

Recalls Dudrick, "We had meetings every day at four o'clock while we were developing that department. It was Ted and Red and me. And we asked Ted to be our representative at M. D. Anderson, and I asked Jim to be our representative primarily in the emergency room and critical care area at Hermann, and I would handle the rest of Hermann and the medical school. We tried to divide up primary responsibilities realistically—although we all had to know about everything. And then at the end of the day, we'd report to each other."[14]

"The collaboration was there and the camaraderie was there," said Gilbert Castro, a researcher down the hall from Red. Moreover, he liked the surgeons: "Surgeons are fun to be with and believe they can do anything." There was an air of "limitless, boundary-less" aspiration.[15] Recollection of those days revived an old excitement in Red, even when he was confined to a wheelchair. "I am telling you, those first years were—oh, I loved them! Everybody was gung-ho, starting something new, and everybody was pulling the wagon. I am talking about the school as well as the department."[16]

Cheves Smythe in planning the building had deliberately put clinical and basic science departments with common interests in proximity to each other. In this way Red's new office in the surgery department on the fourth floor was down the hall from the department of physiology, whose faculty was equally interested in nutrition and metabolism. Smythe's canny design encouraged creative, productive shoptalk across departments and promoted collegiality.

The medical school's first team of surgeons initially planned for Dudrick, Copeland, and Duke to take turns covering the emergency room and trauma service at Hermann Hospital every third night. But when Ted Copeland offered to take over a vacancy in surgery at M. D. Anderson, increased responsibility for the emergency room fell to Duke and Dudrick, who were now covering it every other night instead of every third night. For Red this often became every night, since his chairman was in demand at medical schools and hospitals across the country to present his work on hyperalimentation. And this occurred at a time when Hermann Hospital administration wanted to expand the hospital's trauma service and burn capabilities.

The extra time Red gave the emergency room was time taken away from Betty and the children. For Red, the choice was essentially a question of triage. The patients needed him more. Copeland would tell William Henry Kellar and Heather Green Wooten that "seldom have two men and their families done so much to launch the career of a young academic surgeon. For the next ten years, I had what I considered the best job in American surgery, running a medical school service at the M. D. Anderson Hospital, a category-one cancer institution."[17]

For Red, working around the clock was not a problem, except for

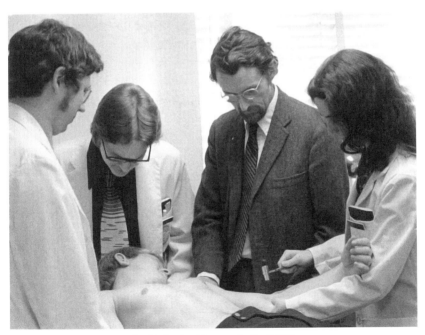

Red teaching at the UT Medical School at Houston in the 1970s.

the shortened time with his family. He did not mind the work. But his children were growing up fast. In a few years Hank would graduate from Memorial High School on the west side of Houston where the family lived. One day at home Hank announced that his Houston high school was the tenth school he had been enrolled in during his lifetime. This was a reminder to Red of how hectic his family's life had been over the years. Similarly, Sara recalls that by high school she had attended a different school nearly every year of her scholastic career. And time at home kept growing shorter as Red's hours in the medical school and the hospital grew longer.

"I did whatever was needed. It was simply my job," he would say, looking back. Work, as his father had taught him, was the unquestionable norm. He doubled down on his efforts, confident that he could overcome any challenge.

"People forget how much vascular and burn surgery I did in the early days," he said. "I loved it, but the demands of the job moved in the direction of trauma care, and I was happy to step in and have a hand in that as well." As it happened, it was through what he did for trauma care at Hermann that Red would make a national name. "When I came in 1972, I have to admit I had no idea why Mr. John Dunn put a heliport on the roof of Hermann Hospital's emergency room. I am ashamed to say, I never asked him why he did it."[18]

In due time Red Duke would find out why, and he would take a leading role in launching the first air ambulance service in Texas, the second in the nation.

CHAPTER 13
Life Flight

Life was good for Steve Dunn the weekend of March 2, 1963. Spring had arrived, and in Texas the bluebonnets painted the countryside as the winter frost gave way to sunny days and warm weather. In Washington, President John F. Kennedy had no idea that in eight months he would be in Texas himself. These were America's Camelot years, and all seemed right with the world.

For Steve Dunn, everything was falling into place. He was twenty-three, a college graduate, a fraternity brother, and now he was attending the University of Texas law school in Austin. His father, John Dunn, was a highly respected and successful businessman in Houston. He was a man of character who was active on community boards and was generous in service to the city. On this weekend Red Duke was in Dallas on call at Parkland. In time Red would find himself in Houston working with John Dunn to change trauma care in that city and across the state as a result of the events about to unfold.

Steve Dunn and his buddies decided to go to Sweetwater—there was a rattlesnake hunt on. Sweetwater claims the largest rattlesnake roundup in the nation, and since 1958, thousands have been attracted to the annual spring ritual with its carnival-like atmosphere, which includes trade stalls, food, rides, and an opportunity to participate in the nervous excitement (and danger) of being in proximity to so many poisonous reptiles.

"For us," Steve said, "it was just another reason to party and not study." After all, what better way for a group of frat boys to enjoy a spring break than a 250-mile road trip to an event that, serpents aside, included lots of cold beer and pretty girls. But as the day wore on, Steve decided the long drive back might be less agreeable than it had sounded earlier. He decided to scout out a faster way to get home. "At the last minute a friend said there was a plane and I could hitch a ride back to Houston."[1]

A free plane ride direct to Houston's Andrau Airpark on the west side sounded good. But it was a plane Steve never should have boarded. The pilot had apparently set the altimeter incorrectly before takeoff and never knew on landing that he was much closer to the ground than his instruments indicated.

With seven on board, the plane was full. Steve went up front to sit in the cramped cockpit with the pilot. The sky was the more interesting because the weather was wet and foggy. But as they were in final approach to the landing strip at Andrau Airpark, something went horribly wrong.

> One minute I was watching the clouds rushing by. The next I was on the ground. We hit the trees and exploded. As it turns out, the pilot should have never landed at Andrau. He should have gone into Houston Hobby, but his car was at Andrau.
>
> I was wearing cowboy boots and I had a hard time getting out. And so I was hanging over the right engine, so that is why my right side got burned worse. And I finally got out and I was on the ground and the thing I remember more than anything else was that I knew I was in trouble, and I said the words, "God, please bless me." I'm convinced that is the reason I was allowed to live.
>
> We were in the middle of nowhere and I was in deep trouble. And just by sheerest luck, two young men were in a car and they saw the crash. They raced across a lot of acreage, I am told, and my friend David Carothers really helped me out. I knew somehow or another that no one could touch me. And yet we had to walk a long ways, it seemed like, and they were able to separate the barbed wire. Somehow I was able to get through [it]. And these young men . . . got me in the back seat and the next thing I know I was in Spring Branch Hospital, which was the closest hospital. The last thing I remember was, I told the people I have contact lenses. That's when they knocked me out.[2]

The following morning the *Abilene Reporter-News* published the story under the headline "7 Cheat Death in Fiery Crash." Another passenger on board, Michael McCrory, had told the reporter, "All of a sudden there was a tremendous roar. I thought we'd been hit by another airplane. The flames were everywhere after we hit, and we couldn't get the back door open. The pilot was burned and bleeding. He kicked open the hatch and we all scrambled out. Steve was running out across the pasture and he was on fire. I ran and tackled him and David [Carothers] caught up and we put out the flames."[3]

Steve's father, John Dunn, was on the board of the Methodist Hospital in Houston's Texas Medical Center and wanted to get his son transferred there from the smaller suburban hospital for the advanced care he would need. There was serious doubt that Steve would survive the transfer, but it had to be attempted. His odds were even worse without specialized care. Every turn, every bump in the road of the fifteen-mile drive sent shockwaves of pain through his body, accompanied by screams of agony. For both father and son, it was unbearable.[4]

Steve survived. John Dunn, traumatized by his son's horrific screams, vowed that day to find a better way to move severely injured patients

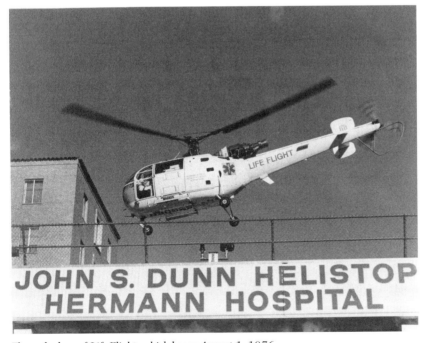

The early days of Life Flight, which began August 1, 1976.

across the city. He looked to the sky for answers. On that day Life Flight, the first air ambulance service in Texas, was born.

John Dunn was a highly respected man in Houston. He was a banker, civic-minded, highly connected, and highly motivated. During the next decade, as his son slowly recovered, Dunn thought about a better way to get severely injured people to the emergency room—it could be done by helicopter. His voice carried weight, and he was willing to put money into his vision of a helicopter racing his son, and others in pain and peril, to care.

In the early 1970s, Dunn gave Hermann Hospital $135,000 to build a heliport atop the hospital's emergency room.[5] Red Duke had just arrived in Houston from Afghanistan. "It was a six-figure number," Steve Dunn says, "which back then was quite a bit of money—I know it was quite a bit of money for my dad. And he said, 'I'll do the heliport and I'll let you all look into how we run it.'" Steve recalls that his father took an instant liking to Red Duke and never had a doubt—this was the right man with the organizational and medical skills to get the job done. John Dunn would remain on the ground and behind the scenes supporting Red Duke's efforts to make one man's dream a life-saving reality for the whole community.

The concept of using air ambulances dates back to 1866, shortly before the Wright brothers were born. It took the imagination of Jules Vern in his 1866 novel *Robur le Conquérant* to describe the rescue of shipwrecked sailors by an airship, a balloon named the *Albatross*.[6] There is a dispute about when air ambulances were first used in the real world. Some say it was at the Siege of Paris in 1870,[7] but more likely, it was during the First World War.

Thanks to the Wright brothers, balloons were outclassed by airplanes in 1903, and three decades later, the world's first practical helicopter, designed by Igor Sikorsky, took flight at Stratford, Connecticut, on September 14, 1939.[8] During the Korean War, when Red Duke was an army tank commander in Germany, the first dedicated use of helicopters by US military forces occurred. It was just a month after the war began that on August 4, 1950, the first rotor wing medical evacuation took place and made history.[9]

The hit television show *M*A*S*H* first aired on September 17, 1972, just weeks after Red Duke joined Stanley Dudrick in Houston.

The popular show depicted the 4077th Mobile Army Surgical Hospital in Uijeongbu, South Korea, and was instrumental in demonstrating the value of the helicopter for saving lives. Each episode began with the famous bubble-fronted Bell 47 rushing wounded soldiers to the waiting scalpels of Benjamin "Hawkeye" Pierce (Alan Alda) and "Trapper John" McIntire (Wayne Rogers).[10] In those days, transport by helicopter was primitive. The wounded were moved on basket stretchers tied to the top of the landing gear, with blankets tied over them. As Red would say, back then, there was nothing for it but to "get them out of harm's way and let God do the rest."[11]

Lives were saved, and many of them. Statistics show that the World War II rate of 4.5 deaths per one hundred casualties dropped to 2.5 during the Korean War, when an estimated twenty thousand injured soldiers were evacuated by helicopter.[12]

Helicopter battlefield evacuation capabilities further improved during the Vietnam War, with larger troop transport helicopters known as Hueys and trained medical evacuation personnel. The televised images were vivid and memorable as night after night Americans watched the evacuation of injured and dead American soldiers from the battlefields of Vietnam. One study noted that soldiers in Vietnam who were evacuated by helicopter with support from medical corpsmen had better rates of survival than motorists injured on California freeways.[13] That success raised the question of how to implement such services for civilians in the United States.

By 1969 the first federal grants were available to assess the impact of medical helicopters on mortality and morbidity in civilian settings, and Mississippi's Project CARE-SOM (Coordinated Accident Rescue Endeavor —State of Mississippi) took the lead with three helicopters purchased through grant funding.[14] The project was considered a success, and it set the stage for the first hospital-based program using a medical helicopter for civilians. In 1972, St. Anthony Central Hospital in Denver, Colorado, obtained an Alouette III helicopter and became a model program with the first hospital-based air ambulance service in the United States.[15]

By the early 1970s, the lessons learned in Vietnam about early evacuation and all-out intensive care of the wounded were increasingly appreciated and were being put into practice in civilian life. Within two years of arriving in Houston, Red Duke, influenced by the evidence out of Vietnam, by what he had seen in the army and in Afghanistan, and also by common sense—in which he specialized—began to create what has become his monument, the Memorial Hermann trauma service.[16] He recalls:

> We started all this probably in early 1973, and somewhere along in 1973 Mr. Dunn built the heliport over the emergency room entrance at Hermann Hospital. . . . It seemed like a good idea, and the whole idea about the helicopter is not any leap of genius. It kind of makes sense—the sooner you can deal with a problem, particularly if it involves bleeding, the better your chance of getting a good outcome. It's called the "golden hour," and that is the time to get trauma care, when the odds are in your favor. Care rendered in that first hour is critical to success- ful outcomes, and the helicopter bought us valuable time.[17]

Some say that care rendered in the golden hour increases chances of survival as much as 80 percent.[18]

Red had heard about an airborne ambulance service in Loma Linda, California. He went there to check it out, but was not impressed; it was, he said, a "rattle-trap" sort of affair. Then Houston deputy fire chief Whitey Martin told him about a service he had heard of at St. Anthony Hospital in Denver. Red and Whitey together approached Bill Smith, a young administrator at Hermann, in a meeting Red said he would never forget. Smith was won over and sent him to Denver.

But to his surprise, Red's reception in Denver was cool. The hospi- tal was not anxious to share information other than the name of the company it rented helicopters from, and it gave Red an impression of wanting to protect its territory. St. Anthony was using the name "Flight for Life" for its program, and when Red asked if Hermann could use the name too, the answer was no.

Red was quick to give Bill Smith credit for getting him out of the starting gate. "He was way ahead of his time. He convinced the board to let us have six months' worth of money to lease the helicopter [and] enough pilots to be safe."[19]

The first helicopter, an Alouette III leased from Rocky Mountain Helicopters, arrived in May of 1976. The lease agreement provided the mechanics, the pilots, and the helicopter. How the helicopter was to be used was left up to Red. In 1975 he gathered a team of three to join him in a small room behind the hospital cafeteria to write protocols, day after day, in preparation for the helicopter's arrival. "We wrote protocols for everything. For the flight crews, for the medication stuff, for the safety on the pad, the development of LZs [landing zones], because there were none."[20] Red's army service had prepared him for organizing big projects with timelines and protocols. Lessons he had learned from preparing instructional materials for the army he now applied to the fledgling endeavor.

One position on the team had to be created from scratch, so Red went to work to create a job description for "flight nurse." "There is no recipe that I know of, there certainly wasn't one then, but we had to figure out how we were going to do this, so we chose several really good ICU nurses and some ER nurses, and we conducted our education program there in the emergency room."[21] Flight nurses would have to assume more responsibility than they were used to in a hospital setting, since they would be working without oversight. Their decision-making in the field would require more knowledge and skill; lives would be directly in their hands. The interns on the flights would know less than a good nurse. There would be no trauma surgeons to fall back on until the patient was evacuated and delivered to the hospital.

The agreement for the helicopter's lease was signed in late winter 1976, with only three months to finalize all the planning and protocols before it arrived in May. Since the Denver program had declined to share its name, "Flight for Life," Red and his team started a contest in the hospital. The winning entry was submitted by a hospital employee. Red, his team, and the hospital administration all liked the name—it was short, simple, and to the point: "Life Flight." It was similar to the name of the Denver program, but, everyone thought, even better.

With protocols written and practice and flight nurses trained, Red had yet another task. "[The nurses] wanted backup, which is natural," he said. "They were pioneers. You've got to admire them. So, we started flying interns. Now, interns in those days were really more educated than interns today, but interns as a whole do not know much, and it wasn't too many months before it became clear who was the boss. It has always been that the flight nurse is the boss medically. The big boss

is the pilot who says go or no go and makes all those kinds of safety decisions."[22]

The first three flights were made on August 1, 1976. "We took a
deep breath and started," Red said. The next month, there were forty-
five. "Two of the first three flights taught me a lesson that I didn't know,"
he added. "Did you know that a television set can explode and burn?"[23]

Red and the early Life Flight crews learned less fiery lessons daily.
Even before Life Flight launched, Red recognized one issue he should
cut off at the pass. As helicopters rushed the seriously injured to Hermann Hospital from all over the city, how would other hospitals and
caregivers react? Was the new air ambulance providing a service or taking business from others in the medical community? Applying Henry's
salesmanship skills, Red made the case to health care providers around
the city that Life Flight was not a threat, but a benefit to everybody.

"Even before we started I did a lot of public relations work. What
I mean by that, trying to be a good country boy, I was just calling people and meeting them and telling them we are not trying to steal your
patients, we just want, when you've got a tough one, to help you out."[24]

At the end of the first six months of funding, the question on everyone's mind was, would the program be renewed? In a tall downtown
building with panoramic views of the city below, the data from the
first few months of the new program were being presented to a meeting of the hospital's board. The vote was about to be held when, out
of nowhere, Life Flight buzzed by the building on the way back to the
hospital with a patient on board. The dignified board members all
scrambled to their feet and crowded the window as Red sat back and
looked on with delight. It was an impressive sight that no board member
could ignore. The program was extended on the spot, and Red would
never admit whether the flyby was real or staged. He would just grin
and say, "They extended the contract and were willing to gamble a little
bit more."[25]

Life Flight's growing pains were continuous, given the constant
need to expand its services and provide for a city that is today the fourth
largest in the nation. In 1986 the governor of Texas, Mark White, was
in Houston to celebrate the program's tenth anniversary. In its first
decade, Life Flight had flown twenty-eight thousand patients. Two
years later it was recognized as the largest civilian air rescue system in

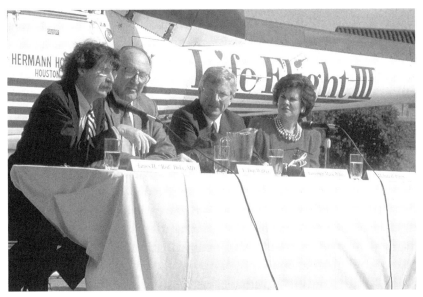

Red Duke at Life Flight's tenth anniversary in 1986. To his left, E. Don Walker, president of the Hermann Trust Administration; Governor Mark White; and Melinda Perrin, Hermann trustee.

the country. In 1983 the original Alouette III helicopters were replaced by three TwinStar helicopters.

On October 23, 1989, near the Houston Ship Channel in Pasadena, a massive explosion rocked a Phillips 66 refinery plant. The fire burned for ten hours and explosions measured 3.5 on the Richter scale. Twenty-three people died that day, and 314 were injured.[26] This marked the first use of Life Flight for a large-scale disaster, and the plans that Red and his team had developed were executed flawlessly. The program repeatedly demonstrated its ability to handle big refinery disasters.

In 2016, Life Flight celebrated its fortieth anniversary and honored Red posthumously for his service as founder and medical director. What had begun as a single leased helicopter had grown by that time into a fleet of six EC-145 twin-engine helicopters and a fixed-wing aircraft, operating on five bases across the Houston area, and serving all the communities within a 150-mile radius of the Texas Medical Center.

During the early years, "we flew by line of sight," one pilot from the 1990s told me. "If we were told the accident was near a red barn off a certain road, we looked for the red barn. We always had to be on the watch for power lines and cables, a problem I rarely had to deal with when flying in Vietnam. Flying at night and in bad weather made it all the more complicated from a safety perspective."[27]

Red and his team worked with the military to bring state-of-the-art technology on board, including night goggles, dual autopilots, weather radar, dual GPS units, 3X color moving-map displays, terrain-and obstacle-warning systems, traffic-avoidance systems, and XM satellite aviation weather monitoring.[28]

Years after founding the program, standing on the impressive heliport on top of Hermann, high above the streets of the Texas Medical Center and a world away from that original helipad atop the old hospital emergency room, Red could often be seen looking to the sky as Life Flight approached with yet another patient. "Ain't she pretty? She's just beautiful!" he would proclaim to anyone who could hear him over the roar of the approaching aircraft. His scrubs and white coat would blow wildly in the wash of the approaching rotors. Just as he had once commanded big tanks with destructive capabilities, he was now at home

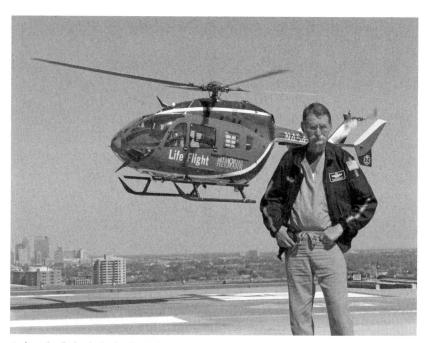

Red on the flight deck of Life Flight.

commanding big helicopters, but their purpose was to save rather than take lives. He loved big challenges and big solutions. Jan Jarboe Russell of *Texas Monthly* said, "Red Duke's theory is that flight crews are like all emergency room personnel: foolish crusaders who are addicted to cheating death. 'They seek out these jobs because of who they are to begin with,' [Duke] said, 'and then this environment we operate in keeps us all hooked.'"[29]

The culture Red and his team created over the years was familial and comradely—rather like that of the army platoons he led while driving tanks through Germany in the early 1950s. Before his death, the pilots honored him in their own way by applying to the Federal Aviation Administration for a "Red Duke" call sign. Such signs are to be used when flying under instrument flight rules (IFR). Now the constant chatter between the pilot and Air Traffic Control when flying IFR is peppered with the identification call "Red Duke." With the call sign approved, Red was taken on board for a ride just a year before his health began to fail. Upon hearing his name repeated throughout the flight in the communication between pilot and control tower, Red could only blush with delight—and allow that he'd never heard his name called out so many times since grade school. It was a moment of undisguised childlike pleasure in knowing that his name would always be assigned to the program he had built, and that the call "Red Duke" would always be associated with saving human lives.

During its first four decades, the program flew 150,000 missions, logging nearly two million miles in the air. At Red's death, Life Flight operations employed a staff of seventy-four, with 80 percent of them having prior military experience.[30] It continues to serve as a model for programs across the country and has been portrayed in three television shows, including a docudrama. Even NASA astronauts have looked to Life Flight for training.

When honored for his founding role and four decades of leadership, Red Duke always deflected the credit to his team—the pilots, flight nurses, paramedics, and support crew. "People have no idea what they face. When they are starting an IV, they may be starting it in a ditch in the middle of the night, upside down. . . . I am very fortunate to come along at a time where I could be involved to some degree in some of the development of this, but I do not take any individual credit."[31]

What he was willing to take credit for was the program's safety record. Only one fatal crash has occurred during the first forty years. On July 17, 1999, a Life Flight helicopter carrying a crew of three crashed just outside Houston while landing to refuel. All three perished. The crash was attributed to a defective part that caused the main rotor blade to detach.[32] The three lost crew members were never far from Red's mind up to the day he died. Their names are memorialized in the hospital's flight operations center, which has evolved from a single red phone on a nurse's triage desk to a state-of-the-art flight control center with technology unimaginable in the early planning.

Safety for his team was Red's first concern, since many of the worst emergencies occur late at night in poor weather. He was not willing to sacrifice his crew members in heroics doomed in advance by weather. Eric von Wenckstern, who was a pilot with Life Flight in its early years and now serves as its administrative director, recounted Duke's advice about whether or not to fly in perilous weather: "We didn't shoot 'em. We didn't stab 'em. We didn't tell them to drink that alcohol and get in

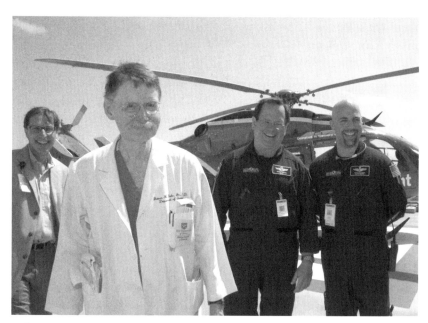

Red Duke with (left to right) Eric Vonwenckstern, director of aviation services; Bobby Wisdom, pilot; and Chivas Guillote, flight nurse, April 1, 2010. Courtesy of Dwight C. Andrews.

their car and crash into a pole, so if you don't think it is safe, don't go."[33]

With that first gift to build a heliport, John Dunn had turned his son's near fatal tragedy into a program to help save thousands of others. It was just the kind of Good Turn that Red Duke admired and wanted to build on. A few months after Red's death, Steve Dunn reflected on the trauma surgeon who had redeemed the senseless tragedy of the night he had nearly died. "Every time I saw him in subsequent years I reminded him of what I had been told about him. I had been told he was a gifted surgeon, a gifted doctor, an extraordinary man, and he was all of those things. . . . It was just a gift from God that a man with his abilities would see and take advantage of the opportunities. And just look at what he has done."[34]

Building a civilian air ambulance program that was a model for communities around the country was one monument in Red Duke's medical career, as Dean Cheves Smythe remarked in his memoirs. But another one was to come.

In 1986 a press conference was held in a Hermann Hospital parking lot to celebrate the tenth anniversary of Life Flight. A Life Flight helicopter loomed behind Red dramatically as, seated at a cloth-draped table, he addressed the audience before him. Texas governor Mark White sat nearby, and print and broadcast reporters pressed close to capture the full story behind the program's local success, which Red summarized as he regaled the crowd.

Red loved an audience, always had something to say, and said it with memorable flair. He was folksy, entertaining, and riding the wave of success. The governor was impressed but not satisfied with what one trauma surgeon in one city had accomplished. Life Flight was a great victory for the Houston area and the Texas Gulf Coast, but what the governor had in mind was a comprehensive, statewide approach to trauma care. He recognized the merit of organizing Texas into regions that could work together across all 254 counties in times of emergency.

Several months after the press conference, Red found himself in Dripping Springs, a small town near Austin, at a wedding reception. Someone had urged him to climb a hill to watch the sun go down over Onion Creek. He did, and among other guests on the hilltop was James A. Michener. Red recognized him and introduced himself, and the two fell into conversation about Afghanistan, the site of Michener's novel *Caravans*.

> And then John Henry Faulk, the radio show host and story-teller, walks up. He was on McCarthy's list with the communism scare back in the '50s. . . . [Faulk] comes up there and says to Michener, "Jim, how are you?" and Mr. Michener says, "I'm fine, Johnny, how are you?" and went back to talking to me. We were just sitting there on a rock. Well, in a little while, Governor White shows up. It turns out we're on his land by his permission. He said, "Red, I didn't think anybody could intimidate John Henry, but you have." He said he came back down there and said, "Those bastards won't talk to me. They're talking about Afghanistan."
>
> And then, out of the clear blue sky—I didn't know a politician knew the words—"Would you help me develop a regionalized trauma system in Texas?" So we started. He created a task force and gave me the money.[35]

During the next legislative session, Red and his task force created a trauma system for the state by organizing its 254 counties into twenty-two groups. He enlisted the chief nurses of Hermann Hospital and Houston's two county hospitals to provide the impetus. Behind the scenes he wrote more than six hundred letters to emergency medical services to be sent under the auspices of the three hospitals.

> Later on we got as many people together as we could and met in the second floor medical school lecture hall, and man, they got organized. . . . It was the damndest thing you ever saw. . . . People don't realize how dedicated and committed these EMS people are. . . . And after 9/11 a lot of money started flowing in. It was first called the Trauma Regional Council, and because we were so efficient, literally the only organized structure in the area during Tropical Storm Allison [the 2001 tropical storm which produced floods that devastated Houston and the Texas Medical Center], the Texas Legislature made them take the word "trauma" out and now we also include stroke and heart attack, so it's a blanket—not just trauma.[36]

Today the Regional Advisory Councils (RACs) are the administrative bodies responsible for trauma system oversight within the bounds of a given Trauma Service Area in Texas. Each of the twenty-two RACS in Texas is responsible for putting together its own functional system. The RACs are structured differently, but they all have the same objective: to reduce the incidence of trauma.[37] Education about trauma and especially trauma prevention was always high on Red's priority list. When he was not in the operating room, he could often be found kicking his cowboy boots against a stool outside one of the busy trauma rooms of the hospital or sitting close to the coffee pot in Life Flight's control center haranguing on his favorite subject—the crisis of trauma-related injuries.

Colleagues recall that he was not bashful about letting his displeasure with politicians be known to anyone within earshot. "To judge by the state budget," he would grouse, "trauma doesn't even exist. No state money goes to pay for treating trauma. Everybody talks about the elephant, feeds it, and cleans up after it, but nobody really sees it or does anything."[38]

His indignation was not without sympathizers. In 1966, the National Academy of Sciences published a report titled *Accidental Death and Disability: The Neglected Disease of Modern Society.* The report was a national wake-up call to the need for research into causes and treatment of traumatic injuries, better education and training of emergency providers, and public and governmental support. A major recommendation was that a professional organization be created to educate the public about trauma and injury prevention.[39] That report was a call to arms for Red Duke and others who believed with him that trauma could be prevented. He became a founding member of the American Trauma Society, which was instrumental in building EMS trauma systems across the country.

While preaching from the pulpit never appealed to Red, preaching about injury prevention and staying healthy came naturally. With his down-home, folksy approach, he would build a syndicated television following in the 1980s that would tune in from coast to coast for some practical medical advice and a good dose of common sense.

CHAPTER 14

TV Doc

Back in the early 1960s, while Red Duke was still in medical school in Dallas, Grant Taylor, who headed pediatrics at M. D. Anderson Hospital (he was "director" then; the title is "chair" now), was pioneering innovative ideas about television to improve both professional and lay access to medical information. In his memoirs, *Remembrances & Reflections*, Taylor mentions a program introduced in South Carolina to connect the public schools electronically, enabling them to share instructional videotapes and thus widen the curriculum without increasing the teaching load.[1]

Taylor was intrigued. What he wanted to link was hospitals across the growing Texas Medical Center. He obtained a copy of a South Carolina instructional videotape and went to work:

> I arranged for the tape to be transmitted from the University of Texas Dental Branch, and for the signal to go by inter-institutional cable to the M. D. Anderson Hospital and, thence, by cable which I strung from lamppost to lamppost across the center, then through an open window on the third floor of the library building, and finally, to the projection equipment on the podium in the auditorium of the library where the Executive Committee of the Harris County Medical Society eagerly awaited their first look at televised medical education.[2]

As the learned audience assembled, Taylor checked and rechecked his signal and was greeted with a clear picture sure to impress the skeptical crowd. But to his dismay, as he took the podium, he heard a loud puck, and the television screen fizzled into a cloud of snowflakes. The unimpressed audience shook their collective heads, and teleconferencing took a back seat as a good idea whose time had not yet come.

Taylor soon learned that a small transistor costing five cents had shorted out and was the sole culprit. "For the next several years," he said, "just as a reminder, I carried the remains of that failed transistor in my wallet."[3] It reminded him never to give up, and he never did. In 1976, while Red was writing protocols to create Life Flight, Grant Taylor's plan to string cable across the Texas Medical Center had evolved far beyond an experimental idea. Eventually Taylor would help launch a Texas Medical Center television network called UT-Television (UT-TV) that in the 1980s and 1990s would produce and syndicate *Dr. Red Duke's Health Reports* worldwide. It broadcast live medical consultations, surgical procedures, and international teleconferences globally.

In the early days of UT-TV, the program's small staff operated out of the medical school, just three floors below Red's office. Although the program had little equipment and only fledgling capabilities, the small cadre of talented staff were more than capable. All they lacked was a big idea, and the president of the UT Health Science Center had that. Mark Carlton, a medical film maker and producer who was a recent addition to the Texas Medical Center, remembers that what Roger Bulger, president of the Health Science Center, wanted was "a fully functional television operation that could serve the entire . . . center." Bulger wanted Carlton to take the present system apart and replace it with a centralized one. "And he wanted it to add health-related programming that would be of service to the community." At the time, such programming was broadcast on weekends in the middle of the night in doses an hour long. What Carlton wanted was something shorter, more frequent, and more accessible. He knew how to get it, too. "News operations were then known as news, weather, and sports," he said. "I wanted them to be known as news, weather, sports, and health information."[4] It was a supremely simple solution.

President Bulger recommended Red Duke to deliver the health segment. Carlton was new enough that he had never heard of Red Duke. He was already intending to syndicate the program, and having the experience of working with West Coast professionals, he wanted someone with name recognition. But, despite his misgivings, he consented to go to Duke's office, look him over, and give him a screen test.

"When I arrived," Carlton reports, "he was playing Willie Nelson music so loud I could hardly carry on a conversation with him, and then he would stop and sing along once in a while, which was pretty fun, I guess, but I was trying to get a point across to him. When I finally did get my point across about what the president had talked about, he looked at me and [said], 'If the chief thinks I can do it, let's run the flag up and see if anyone salutes.'"[5]

With that, Red Duke the surgeon was about to become Red Duke the syndicated TV doc. A thirty-minute pilot was planned and a script written in coordination with the health science center's communication team, including Joe Siegler and Don Macon. Red, who had never done television work other than interviews with local media, looked the script over and felt that with a couple of readings he could do it. Mark Carlton picks up the story:

> So Greg [West] takes Dr. Duke on top of what was a parking garage with the background of the medical center behind him. He shot this little pilot, with Red saying, "You know, there are forty thousand people working in this medical center to help take care of you in emergencies and to help you have better health." Then he [did] a little segue into some report about some health topic. This first program was thirty minutes in length, and had about five of those little segments in it. So that was our pilot.
>
> I took that over to Channel 13 and the programming directors viewed it and said, "Wait a minute. Stop the presses. We have to have someone come in and see this." So they went down, got a bunch of news people to come in. They said, "This is the way you need to be shooting television news." And I said, "Well, what about my project? Do you think it has some possibilities? What do we need to do to change it? Is there anything we need to do to polish it?" "Don't touch it. Don't touch it. We want to air this as it is, and we have a thirty-minute time slot open on Friday night at a certain date ahead, and we would like to air it at that time." And then they dropped the bombshell. They said, "But the cost is twenty thousand dollars for that time spot." Remember, this was 1981. So it was twenty thousand dollars for that entire half-hour time, and I said, "We are willing for you to use the program, but the twenty thousand dollars has to come from somewhere else."[6]

Where to get twenty thousand dollars? Soon Carlton was meeting with Matt Provenzano, the president of Texas Commerce Medical Bank (later the Texas Commerce Bank). After they had viewed the pilot, Carlton asked Provenzano if his bank wanted to sponsor part of the program. "Part of it? I want the whole half hour."

The program aired and the station's phone lines lit up all night and into the next day. People wanted more. They liked this cowboy surgeon who was a straight talker and entertaining to watch. In time, three more half-hour programs were developed before refining the idea to make them into smaller, ninety-second health segments that could be integrated into the news.

The formula worked, and *Texas Health Reports* featuring Red Duke from the University of Texas Health Science Center at Houston was soon syndicated from coast to coast, including to the US military network worldwide. Recalls Carlton, "I would take samples to a local market and show each station a clip and tell them by the end of the day, whichever station acted first, that would be the station to get the program for their market. My travel schedule frequently meant five cities in five states in five days. I visited them all."[7]

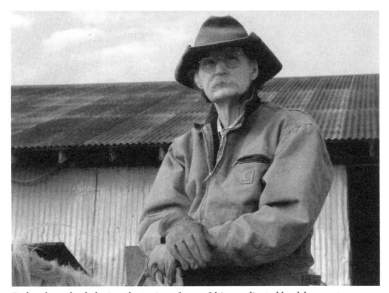

Red on horseback during the taping of one of his syndicated health reports.

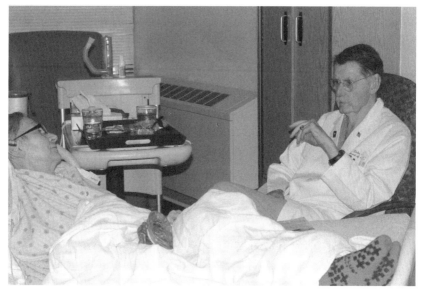

Red visiting a patient. "Who's the most important person in the room?" Red would ask his students. Always, the patient.

Red Duke could discuss a health topic from head to toe, give commonsense advice about it, and keep his audience reminded that "accidents don't just happen." He would don a construction hard hat and take a jackhammer to a street corner to illustrate advances in breaking up kidney stones using ultrasound, a procedure called lithotripsy. Another segment might find him on horseback, the spitting image of an old West trail hand at the end of a long, dusty cattle drive, who charges his mount head-on toward his destination—in Duke's case, the camera—with something important on his mind: "You know, it's real easy to be judgmental of other folks, but always remember, we are all imperfect, flawed souls susceptible to all types of dangerous behavior—addictions being a classic example—all of which can cause harm. One of the most tenacious of all addictions is smoking."[8]

Each segment was written by Red with precision and his personalized no-nonsense approach. Many of the messages came from "sitdowns" with his patients. Sit-downs were famous among his many residents who followed him around on late-night hospital rounds. If there was an empty chair, Red would sit down and spend some time. It was a lesson he insisted his students learn and adopt: physicians treat people, not diseases.

Red Duke's sit-downs were notorious. It was not uncommon for residents and fellows rounding with Red late at night to remove a bedside chair from a room before Red arrived, to keep him from sitting down and regaling the patient with stories and conversation late into the night. Red's message to his students on patient rounds was to slow down and spend quality time with the patient. Students understood that the patient was always the most important person in the room, no matter what hour of the day or night it was. What they questioned was when Red ever found time to sleep.

The success of *Texas Health Reports* had unexpected reverberations. Red Duke was known and loved everywhere, including in Hollywood. Interest in him there generated the idea for an ABC television series, *Buck James*, to star Dennis Weaver. Weaver had played the role of Chester on *Gunsmoke*, a series that was a favorite of Red's. And now Chester of *Gunsmoke* would play Buck James, a character based on Red. The *Buck James* series appeared for a short run during the 1987/1988 season.[9] Red, who always loved to hobnob with celebrities, was more than elated when he was contacted by network producers who wanted Dennis Weaver to go to Houston and shadow him in preparation for the role. In short, Dennis Weaver was to be Red's sidekick for a while.

The two got along famously. Red consulted on scripts with the show's writers and producers while showing Weaver how to act like a surgeon. Weaver scrubbed up and stood behind Red in surgery, absorbing the presence that Red commanded in his world of medicine. Here no make-believe script was needed; the daily drama that sought out a trauma surgeon created its own storylines. As Dennis Weaver was deliberately morphing into Red Duke, who had already taken on a likeness to Weaver's earlier character Sam McCloud, the two could be seen walking the hospital corridors, eerily alike—both tall, angular, and talking with pronounced twangs under big mustaches. They turned heads and created a predictable stir.

Outside the hospital the two would often take in Red's favorite restaurants, including barbecue joints, where the Duke/Weaver duo made a popular sighting. Red loved barbecued ribs and sometimes abandoned his usually healthful fare to indulge in them. As fans pressed in for a

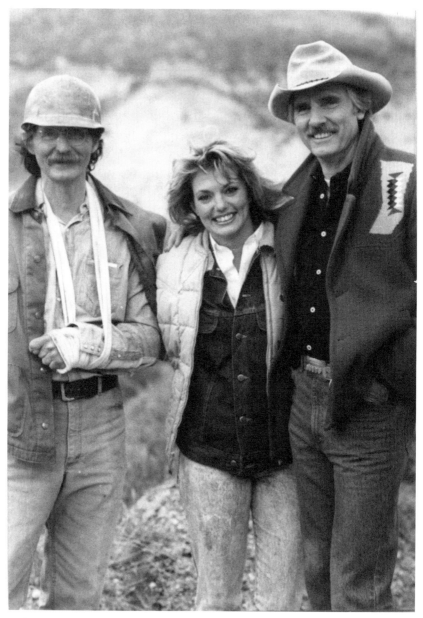

Red and Pam Duke on the set of Buck James with Dennis Weaver in 1988. Red played the role of an injured oil field worker. Courtesy of Pam Duke.

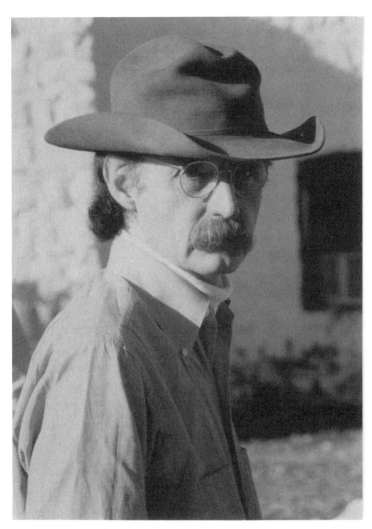

Classic Red Duke in hat.

photo or autograph, few probably noticed that Dennis Weaver was not eating ribs. He was a devout vegetarian.

Red not only prepared Weaver for the role, but also made a cameo appearance in one episode of *Buck James*. He played an oil field rough-neck injured and in need of Weaver's surgical skills. Between takes, Red would step out of his character as patient to offer suggestions in the interests of authenticity. That the series was short-lived and ended after one season was disappointing to Red, but, always practical, he shrugged it off as show business. It was just entertainment, and probably no one had been more entertained than Red Duke, watching Hollywood create its own version of his life in medicine. The show ended, but the thrill of having worked with Dennis Weaver would last a lifetime.

Red's son Hank discusses how Weaver's Sam McCloud character influenced Red Duke's look: "When we returned from Afghanistan in 1972, Dennis Weaver was starring in *McCloud* [1970–77], about a commonsense cowboy marshal from New Mexico on loan to the police in New York City. That show was mandatory viewing in our house, and over time my dad adapted that McCloud look, switching to his gold military-issue wire-rim glasses, growing the mustache and longer hair, and adding the cowboy hat."[10]

It was a look that the public had fallen in love with, and it was probably in no small part responsible for Red Duke's celebrity.

In this way Dennis Weaver and his character Sam McCloud had helped shape Red Duke's public persona and his look, while Red had provided a new role for Weaver to play. The McCloud persona did not of course change Red Duke, who was fundamentally immutable. But it tweaked his look. It made him look more like himself.

NBC's *Lifeline*, a documentary that aired between September 1978 and early 1979, followed the daily routines of some of the most successful doctors in the country. The program featured Red Duke in one episode. Building on his television success, Red hosted the PBS show *Bodywatch*, which aired from 1986 to 1989 and was produced by WGBH/Boston, in association with *American Health Magazine*. National exposure led to more national exposure. Multiple appearances on the national news programs followed along, including *NBC Nightly News*, *The Today Show*, and *PM Magazine*. Red Duke was becoming a household name across the country as newspaper and magazine reporters joined in to feature this cowboy-*cum*-surgeon beloved by the public.

"Hell," Red said of his television work, "I didn't know what I was doing. I just did it. . . . The chairman of the communications school up in Austin once told me, 'Red, I love your stuff. I make the students watch it all the time. You do it all wrong, but it works.'"[11]

What Red did right was be himself and talk to the viewers exactly as he would talk to his patients and his medical students. There in the hospital, the busy trauma unit presented him with an endless stream of health topics that needed talking about, and he had plenty to say. The colleagues who worked alongside him are adamant that he was the same person in the hospital corridors and operating rooms and at the bedside that he was on television. That translates to Red Duke vernacular as "It is what it is."

In 1989, Surgeon General Everett Koop announced his retirement. A serious groundswell of support pushed Red Duke to the forefront as a possible replacement. Susan Ayala, a staff writer for the *Wall Street Journal*, gave the movement a national spotlight with a July 6, 1989, headline: "'Cowboy Doc' Is an Unusual Candidate to Succeed Koop as Surgeon General."

> Every other word is "sumvabitch." He only recently gave up chewing tobacco. And there's talk of making him surgeon general.
>
> Dr. James H. "Red" Duke hardly seems the conventional candidate for the nation's top medical post. His faded jeans, cowboy boots and horse named Socks are straight out of "Lonesome Dove." . . .

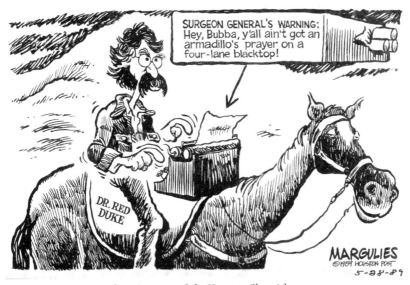

Image by Jimmy Margulies. Courtesy of the Houston Chronicle.

In a real-life operating room, Dr. Duke leans over, ready to remove a patient's gallbladder. A radio plays what he calls the best song in the whole world: "I'm Gonna Hire a Wino to Decorate Our Home." The song is pure country, and that's what Dr. Duke likes. . . .

Now, some local and national health officials and local Republican politicians are involved in a grass-roots effort to send Dr. Duke to Washington to succeed Surgeon General C. Everett Koop, who is retiring. . . .

Chase Untermeyer, a transplanted Houstonian who is assistant to [President George H. W. Bush] and director of presidential personnel, says a list of candidates for surgeon general is being gathered and he's hearing a lot about Red Duke.

. . . Dr. Duke thought the whole surgeon general idea was "a little crazy" at first. But he was convinced "it wouldn't be such a bad idea" though he says he'd hope to work in a little trauma surgery on the side.[12]

While Red's popularity with the general public was a strong point in his favor for acceding to the position of surgeon general, his outspoken contempt for bureaucratic meddling in health policy probably lost him important support in Washington. He was destined to be loved, but he was not destined to be surgeon general.

Red's growing celebrity brought him back in touch with his childhood acquaintance Willie Nelson, who had left Abbott and risen to musical stardom. Red joined Nelson as medical director for the singer's popular July 4 music festivals around Austin. Reporting for the *Austin American-Statesman*, John Bryant summarized Duke's contribution to Willie's upcoming July 4, 1986, Farm Aid II concert near Austin:

Overheated music fans knocked groggy by the summer sun at the Farm Aid II concert July 4 may gaze up into the familiar, reassuring face of Dr. Red Duke. . . . "Willie asked me through his daughter, Lana," said Duke, who flew to Austin Wednesday to revise medical treatment plans that had been fashioned for UT's Memorial Stadium before the concert was moved last week to South Park Meadows. . . .

The country-talking doctor said he and Nelson have been running into each other since the two grew up together in Hill County—Nelson in Abbott and Duke in Hillsboro.

Duke said he has "blown out a lot of speakers and worn out a lot of tape decks" listening to Nelson's country music in his pickup. He even plays Willie Nelson tunes in the operating room of Houston's Hermann Hospital.[13]

When his mother was ill, Willie Nelson asked Red to look in on her. Red was deeply touched by that.

But at times, Red's fame got in his way. One veteran flight nurse in the late 1980s recalls the night of a horrific multicar accident requiring the entire fleet of Life Flight helicopters on the scene. As they rushed to lift off from the hospital's heliport, they were a crew member short, so Red jumped in. On the scene dozens of onlookers and emergency personnel watched anxiously as the helicopter settled gracefully to the ground. But then, as Red stepped out, several onlookers gasped his name. In minutes he was swarmed by the crowd, including several of the walking injured and a few emergency personnel—all anxious to see Red Duke in person. As much as Red's help was needed at the accident scene that night, the stir created by his celebrity made it nearly impossible for him to render aid as a member of the flight team. He didn't try after that. He stayed back at the hospital coordinating the team and tending to patients as they arrived.

The UT-TV production crew, notes Mark Carlton, never had to worry about the quality of Red's scripts or about his performance in front of the camera. What they did have to worry about was getting him in front of the camera at all, since he was occupied around the clock with surgery, seeing patients, and teaching. The ability to bide their time was a virtue the entire film crew learned early. A call from Red might run along these lines: "I've been operating on this police officer for six hours and I'm not done—hang tight." When the surgery was complete, recalls Tom Eschbacher, "we'd typically get a call—'Hi, this is Dr. Duke. Y'all ready to work?'" He adds, "Countless times he told us, 'I love doing this shit with you all.'"[14] The television crew loved him and would have waited all night without complaint.

Eschbacher, a videographer and editor for Red's health reports for ten years, noted that Red never used a teleprompter on camera and needed only a few moments to memorize his script. He said that Duke "loved showing off his TV bloopers, curse words and all. His favorite blooper occurred at the Houston Livestock Show and Rodeo. I had just started recording him standing in front of a large bull when the animal lifted its tail and proceeded to take a dump. At that moment, Dr. Duke looked back at the bull, faced the camera again, and with a huge grin said, 'From the University of Texas Health Science Center at Houston, I'm Dr. Red Duke.'"[15]

For eighteen years Red wrote every script for his *Texas Health Reports*. Boxes of scripts piled up in his office over time, each carefully

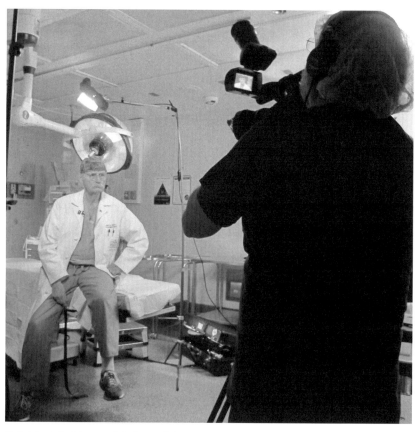

Red doing television work in front of the camera.

printed in his own hand on yellow notepad paper, to be typed up and polished into a production script by the UT-TV writers and producers. Writers like Elaine Mays worked behind the scenes throughout the program's run to fact-check and smooth out any edges. Syndication of the program brought in nearly six million dollars in revenue over the years, notes Carlton, but Red never asked for or expected a penny.[16] The program's revenues helped support the production costs, equipment, and salaries of the team.

Although Red never became surgeon general, in hindsight he could not regret it, because of everything else he had going on during those years—surgery, professional societies, the air ambulance service, teaching, and the business of celebrity. And there was another interest that also competed for his time. It was a passion he had cultivated since his early Boy Scout days and it had absolutely nothing to do with medicine.

CHAPTER 15
A Conservationist at Heart

The Sioux were starving. They had lost their beloved lands to the white man, whose greed seemed boundless. Moreover, the great buffalo herds, which had thundered across the plains in their millions, were rapidly disappearing. Throngs of settlers and bluecoats had been brought by the iron horse across the Indian's treasured hunting grounds, where they had killed thousands upon thousands of buffalo. Often they took only the hide or the tongue and left the great beast to rot where it fell. Sitting Bull must have been sick at heart.

In Dee Brown's classic *Bury My Heart at Wounded Knee*, there is a telling and stunning statistic: "of 3,700,000 buffalo destroyed from 1872 until 1874, only 150,000 were killed by Indians."[1] Plains Indians depended on native game and the buffalo to survive. Their housing, clothing, tools, and other substance, and their spirituality, were all linked directly to the land and the ample resources it had supported, including the wildlife they had respected for centuries, especially the buffalo. Every fiber of the buffalo was a gift from above to be treasured and used for a purpose.

Native American tribes of the Great Plains, including the Crow, Sioux, Cheyenne, Apache, and Comanche, watched the decimation of the buffalo in horror. Their way of life changed abruptly, and they were faced with starvation and removal to designated Indian agencies. Even for Ranald S. Mackenzie, the commanding officer of Fort Sill in the Oklahoma territory, who was not known for tenderness of heart, the plight of the Plains Indians became troubling.[2] They called him "Bad Hand." MacKenzie had made a career of killing Indians, yet in a rare moment of shame, he wrote to his commanding officer, General Philip Sheridan: "I am expected to see that Indians behave properly whom the government is starving—and not only that, but starving in flagrant violation of agreement."[3]

Dee Brown tells the story of one small group of Cheyennes, a remnant of their once great tribe, that Mackenzie "allowed" to leave their agency confinement under watch for a single buffalo hunt to feed their starving families. "The buffalo hunt was so miserable a failure that the hunters would have joked about it, had not everyone been starving for meat. Buffalo bones were everywhere on the southern Plains, ghostly heaps of bones left by white hunters, but the Cheyennes could find nothing to hunt but a few coyotes. They killed the coyotes and ate them, and before the winter was over, they had to eat their dogs, too, to supplement the agency's meager rations of beef."[4]

Red Duke saw the injustices dealt a proud people who for centuries had nurtured the resources they depended on. Red's paternal great-grandmother Nancy Cherry's Cherokee descent connected him through the marrow of his bones with Native Americans and their belief in the necessity for good stewardship of natural resources, including wildlife.

Moreover, Red's greatest hero, Albert Schweitzer, had won the Nobel Peace Prize for his concept of "reverence for life." The phrase was the backbone of an ethical philosophy that Schweitzer, and later Duke, lived by daily. As Schweitzer's biographer, James Brabazon, interpreted it, "We are brothers and sisters to all living things, and owe to all of them the same care and respect that we wish for ourselves."[5] That we owe reverence to life is nevertheless inextricable from the fact that life feeds on life. Schweitzer tried to overcome that troubling contradiction with vegetarianism, at which he succeeded only imperfectly. Duke, however, accepted this inconsistency at the heart of things, and he seems to have had no difficulty marrying reverence for life with hunting, much less with eating.

Wildlife conservation, like medicine, was a calling that blended Duke's heart and head. In the last year of his life, he was presented the Peter Hathaway Capstick Award, which is the Dallas Safari Club's highest and most distinguished award for wildlife conservation. Red had received many awards in his lifetime, but this one was special.

"I was born right before the Great Depression," he said in his remarks to the club on the night of the awards ceremony, "and you learned during those years that whatever you had was precious. When I got older and got involved in wildlife, it was obvious I was just doing what I felt like God wanted me to do. You know God created this unbelievably wonderful world in which we find ourselves and all the other

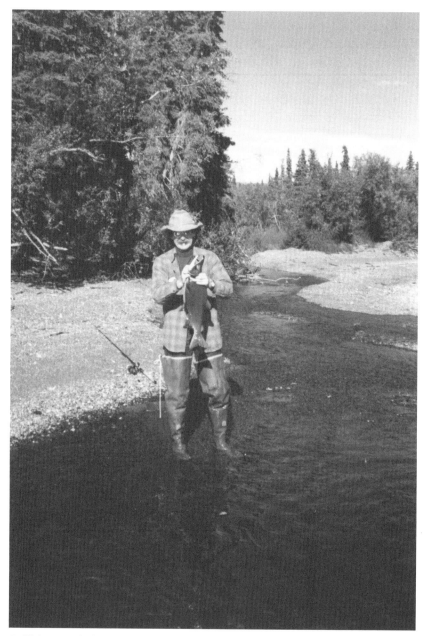

Red fishing in Alaska. Alaska was a special place and held many of his favorite hunting and fishing memories. Courtesy of Pam Duke.

creatures on it. We must learn to take care of it. It's got a finite ability to support reckless use."[6]

Red Duke had always loved the outdoors, and he grew up with a love of hunting and fishing. Far from home in New York as a young army tank commander awaiting orders for Germany, he had written a letter to his mother, wondering how the fishing was at home and lamenting that the worst thing about being away in the fall would be that he could not go deer hunting with his family (October 19, 1951).

Over the years, a growing collection of trophy deer, antelope, elk, and bighorn sheep heads found their way from the taxidermist to Duke's home and office walls. High-elevation trekking for big game was especially challenging and extreme, and therefore especially beloved by Red. Students and colleagues at the medical school could often tell when he was about to leave for a hunting trip in the mountains, because he could be found in the school's gym working out to build the stamina he would need for his upcoming high-altitude adventures.

On one hunting trip to Alaska in September 1979, Red ended up stranded on the Matanuska Glacier in the Chugach Mountains. The pilot, Hank Hankard, had taken another hunter and the guide to a different location and left Red alone on the glacier as a storm set in. It blocked Hank's return for two days. Red and he were both veterans of the remote Alaskan wilderness and were good friends, so Red knew the drill as he awaited the familiar sound of the returning plane. High on the mountain glacier, with a blizzard raging outside, Red secured his gear and hunkered down in his tent. Fortunately he had pen and paper with him. He had learned the hard way to take something to occupy him in just such an event, "because you can get left out there for a long time. . . . I wrote a chapter for a textbook on surgery that I needed to write, and I was late writing it. I didn't have anything else to do so I just wrote that chapter. It actually turned out pretty good."[7]

In 1981, Red acquired an Alaskan assistant-guiding license in order to take charge of his own hunts and guide others across the thrilling, remote Alaskan wilderness that he so deeply loved. Obtaining the license required documentation of his cumulative experience of big game hunting in Alaska and recommendation from a registered guide-outfitter willing to hire his services. Additionally, as an applicant his prior criminal justice information would have been reviewed to ensure

that he held the necessary big game licenses with no outstanding viola-
tions of game laws in any state. One last requirement likely brought a
grin to Red's face—a card attesting to his knowledge of basic first aid.
Once he had passed all the hurdles, Red was assessed license fees annu-
ally to maintain his guide/outfitter status.

For Red Duke, hunting and camping hundreds of miles from the
nearest hospital and civilization was a challenge to be relished. He also
understood that far from civilization in rugged back country lurked
dangers no amount of experience nor medical know-how could provide
protection against, and now, as a guide, he was responsible for others
as well. In these remote stretches, grizzly bears were known to follow
the sound of a gunshot in search of an easy meal (including hunters),
hidden icy crevasses waited to swallow the hapless adventurer, frostbite
came quickly, and falls off steep terrain could prove deadly. The ways to
be injured or worse are many in such frozen wildernesses, and Red relished the chance to match his senses and skills to meet whatever threats
to life and limb came his way.

• • •

Conservation movements in the United States go back to the years
before the Civil War, when a handful of people who loved hunting and
the outdoors began to speak out about managing habitat and wildlife
for the enjoyment of future generations.

The disappearance of the buffalo became a rallying cry for those who
first signaled concern about the future of wildlife in the United States.
The demise of the passenger pigeon added another layer of alarm. In
1813 James Audubon, the famous artist and ornithologist, reported
sighting a flight of passenger pigeons in one day that stretched fifty-five
miles and contained an estimated one billion birds. The last passenger
pigeon died in the Cincinnati Zoo in 1914, almost four decades before
Red Duke visited that zoo in June 1951 on one of his army weekend
forays from officer training at Fort Knox.[8]

In 1842 the US Supreme Court denied a landowner's claim to
exclude others from taking oysters from some mudflats in New Jersey.
That case, *Martin v. Waddell*, codified the concept that in the United
States all wildlife and fish belong to all the people and that the stewardship of those fauna is entrusted to the individual states.[9]

The Civil War put a dent in the progress being made in respect to conservation movements, but thanks to an outspoken advocate with an apt name, George Bird Grinnel, conservation took on a new life after the war ended. Grinnel wrote numerous articles in his magazine, *Forest and Stream*, about the plight of US forests and wildlife, and people listened, including a twenty-three-year-old Harvard graduate and member of the New York legislature who went on his first buffalo-hunting trip in 1883. Theodore Roosevelt, an avid outdoorsman and hunter, was shocked to find no buffalo where once there had been vast herds blanketing the plains. They were gone, and he was furious.

When Roosevelt's wife, Alice, and his mother, Mittie, died only a few hours apart on February 14, 1884, Roosevelt, although he was a well-respected politician with a busy life in the city, felt that he needed to get back to the outdoors. He returned to the Badlands of North Dakota for three years to reflect on his life and establish his beloved Elkhorn Ranch.[10] There he would ride the fence lines for days and work as one with the cowboys as they herded cattle and hunted the open plains.

With his bushy mustache, wire-rimmed glasses, and bigger-than-life presence, the former Boy Scout Teddy Roosevelt bore some resemblance to Red Duke. Roosevelt too loved trophies and harbored a spiritual kinship with nature. And of course they shared a passion for conservation. "The nation behaves well," Roosevelt said, "if it treats the natural resources as assets which it must turn over to the next generation increased and not impaired in value. Conservation means development as much as it does protection."

Teddy Roosevelt would become the most active president in the history of American conservation, setting aside 230 million acres during his presidency. He presided over the creation of eighteen national monuments, fifty-one wildlife refuges, four national game preserves, and five national parks.[11]

In addition, in 1887 Roosevelt gathered a group of influential American hunters in New York City to form the Boone and Crockett Club, whose mission was to preserve the big game of North America. It is America's oldest conservation club. Through Roosevelt, the Boone and Crockett Club gave rise to the "fair chase" concept, which specifies that game must be born in the wild (as opposed to being bred in captivity and released for the hunt) and may not be confined for the hunt. Failure to observe that rule has given rise to canned hunts, at which sometimes virtually tame animals are held in pens to be shot effortlessly.

In his time Red Duke was to become a member of the Boone and Crockett Club. He was active in the organization and served on editorial and historical committees, and committees on ethics, communications, strategic planning, and awards. In 1984 he received a call from the club's president asking him to consider leading the organization.

> We were coming up on the centennial of Boone and Crockett. I'd been as active as I could in any way that I knew how when I got this call. We normally had our big major meeting on the first Wednesday and Thursday of December. Well, I got this call on Tuesday from Bill Spencer. Spencer was the president and CEO of Citibank in New York. . . . He said, "I want you to be president of Boone and Crockett," and I was taken aback— and I said, "I'm gettin' ready to be president of the Foundation for North American Wild Sheep," which was true, in January, and he said, "I know it." Like he really cared! He was not in the habit of—you know, the president of Citibank doesn't ask for a discussion! It's just ordered, and so I became president.
>
> [It was] January '86, I guess, and we were meeting over at Johnny Hanes' house in Alexandria [Virginia]—you've heard of Hanes Hosiery? His family is big owners in Winchester and that sort of stuff. A buddy walked in and said that the Challenger just blew up. So I was a little busy that year, and this damn TV got started. I was doin' that then, too. I don't know how I did all that stuff.[12]

During his tenure as president, Red worked with the board on a number of big projects, including buying the Theodore Roosevelt Memorial Ranch, located near Dupuyer, Montana. The Boone and Crockett foundation was formed as well, and charged with managing the six thousand acre property to conduct habitat research, conservation education programs, and land management demonstrations. This effort included collaborating with the University of Montana to oversee the research aspects of the program and create a Boone and Crockett wildlife professorship there.

Another Boone and Crockett initiative under Red's presidency included publishing an associates' newsletter focusing on hunting and conservation articles. By 1994 the newsletter would become the organization's quarterly magazine, *Fair Chase*.

Indeed, as president, Red was active on multiple fronts during his tenure, continually drawing from his committee service over the years and the experience he had gained through other conservation groups he had served, including the Foundation for North American Wild Sheep.

Red was president of Boone and Crockett for four years (1985–89), including the organization's centennial year in 1987. As he was about to go out of office, one item on his agenda remained unfinished. The club wanted to build a log cabin in the Buffalo Bill Center of the West, located in Cody, Wyoming. It would be devoted to American firearms, and one member, Bill Ruger, had donated a million dollars to the cause. But more money was needed to get the project settled.[13] Deliberations about how to raise it had proved fruitless, and Red did not want to go out of office with a failure on his hands.

The last board meeting of Red's presidency took place in Chicago at the Field Museum. Red had arranged for the dinner to be served very slowly. Within easy reach of the diners, a long table had been set up with bottles of scotch, bourbon, and wine. When the speaker sat down, Red addressed the table. "'Gentlemen, there's one more thing to do, and that's finish out . . . this cabin [funding]. Now the doors are locked. The police are at the door. We're not going anywhere until we finish it.' And we did."[14]

• • •

About 750,000 years ago, in the Pleistocene era, wild sheep crossed the Bering land bridge from Siberia into Alaska and North America. Within a few hundred thousand years they diverged in North America into several species. In Alaska there are the magnificent Dall sheep. From southern Canada to Mexico, the bighorn sheep evolved over the centuries into at least seven distinct subspecies—the actual number is still in dispute.[15] One of those groups captured Red Duke's attention and dedication—the desert bighorn sheep (*Ovis canadensis nelson*).

Named for the large, curved horns of the rams, the desert bighorns can weigh as much as three hundred pounds. Their agility in climbing

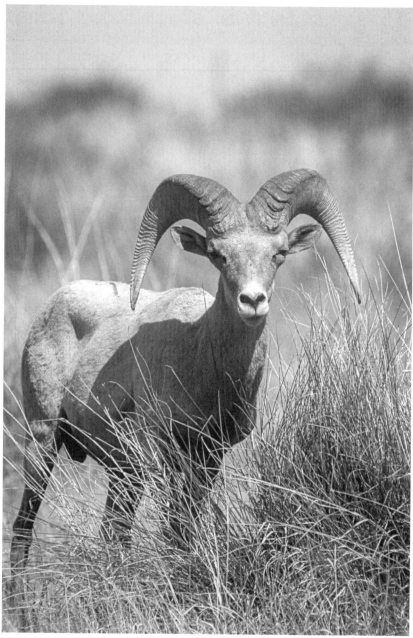

Tagged desert bighorn ram at Sierra Diablo Wildlife Management Area. Courtesy of Texas Parks and Wildlife.

steep, rocky terrain can be spellbinding as they seek cover from predators, including bears, wolves, and especially cougars. Their high-altitude habitat is extreme, and the harder it is to find, the happier they seem to be. They are a creature that was bound to attract the attention and admiration of Red Duke.

By some estimates, in the early 1800s there were more than two million bighorn sheep throughout Canada, the western United States, and northern Mexico. Mountainous tribes of Indians depended on these sheep just as the plains Indians depended on the buffalo, and petroglyphs depicting bighorns number in the thousands throughout their mountainous US range.[16] By 1900 there were only a few thousand of the sheep left, due to hunting, disease, and competition from ranching, but thanks to federal and state-led conservation efforts, the complete demise of the bighorn has been avoided.

No discussion of Red Duke and conservation would be complete without a few stories about his favorite cause, saving the desert bighorn sheep. "Some guys had formed the Foundation for North American Wild Sheep, and I got involved. Well, sheep, to me, are kinda the most majestic and captivating of all the big game, and I started paying more attention to them. Over time it became a passion because they are just so magnificent."[17]

As Colorado had provided Red a model program for starting an air ambulance service, Arizona provided a model conservation project for saving the bighorn sheep. That the Boy Scouts were involved put the story all the closer to Red's heart.

In the 1930s the Arizona Boy Scouts were worried about the demise of the bighorns. At the time there were fewer than 150 bighorn sheep in the state, and a "save the bighorn" poster contest was started by the Boy Scout council in Phoenix, with the winning bighorn emblem to be made into neckerchief slides for the ten thousand Boy Scouts across the state.[18]

The number of bighorn sheep in Texas was also dwindling then, and by the time Red graduated from college in 1950, the small Texas population of desert bighorns in the mountainous regions of West Texas was gone—totally extinct.

Writing for *Texas Parks and Wildlife* magazine in 2016, the department's former communication director, John Jefferson, chronicled the efforts of Red and other concerned Texans in the early 1980s to bring the bighorns back to Texas. Early attempts to restore the sheep, he reported, had foundered on predation. But luck stepped in. Jack Kilpatric, a biologist who worked for the Texas Parks and Wildlife Department (TPWD) and headed the attempt there to reintroduce bighorn sheep into Texas, and Tommy Caruthers, a hunter who had good connections in the state, fell into conversation over empty gas tanks in Marfa. Kilpatric said that the sheep could be reintroduced if there were money for pens to protect them against predation. Caruthers volunteered that he had friends who might be able to help. In short order, the Texas Bighorn Society was formed, and one of those friends, Red Duke, was named its first president.[19]

The group raised nearly two hundred thousand dollars to build new pens on the Sierra Diablo Wildlife Management Area, a remote, mountainous region near Van Horn (120 miles southeast of El Paso), owned and managed by the TPWD. Red recalls:

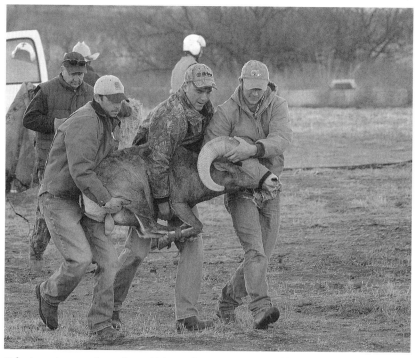

Volunteers transporting a desert bighorn sheep into Sierra Diablo Wildlife Management Area. Courtesy of Texas Parks and Wildlife.

I knew there was an Arizona Bighorn Society, but I had no earthly idea what they did. Well, I got a dozen Texans together, and we started [a bighorn society], and it took about a year to get legal. What I mean by that is a charitable organization, 501(c)(3). Then we agreed to have a meeting with the biologist at that seven-thousand-acre thing that's called the Sierra Diablo—ah, it's gotta title beyond that—it's right at Van Horn. You always gotta have some experts, and in those days the standard was that a guy was an expert if he came from more than two hundred miles away and had a boxful of slides. We had a guy from New Mexico and a guy from California, but we ended up doing what the sheep biologist suggested, since he'd been working with 'em a long time. What we did, and damned if we didn't—we didn't know what we were doin', but we built these four ten-acre brood pastures. They had eight-foot fences around 'em.

Then, we put an eleven-foot fence around that with a hot wire on top . . ., and we didn't have any mountain lion trouble. Then, we gave that to the state, just volunteered. I mean, it was all volunteer stuff. Man, it was so easy to get pipe donated in 1982, because there was a big oil crisis, and this kinda buddy of mine that was in the steel business, I'd send all that pipe to him in Fort Worth. He'd clean it up and send it out there, and he just acted as a general contractor, and we did a lot of that pretty damn cheap.[20]

Red and his friends dug into their pockets to pay for the project, while dreaming up fundraising ideas to get the public involved. One such idea involved a public hanging of Red Duke. John Jefferson, who saw a film of the famous hanging shortly after the event, reported the story three decades later in the October 2016 issue of *Texas Parks and Wildlife* magazine:

At one of their meetings to discuss funding, the idea was floated to have Dr. Red Duke arrested. Organizations were raising money that way, by . . . having alleged perpetrators "arrested," and then requiring them to solicit "bail" money

from their friends. Hearing that, Clayton Williams, a prominent oil and gas operator and accomplished sheep hunter,
readily announced that he would happily pay $16,000 to see
Red Duke go to jail. . . .

The plan then took on a life of its own, getting bigger and
wilder as it went. When Duke got off the plane in Van Horn, he was
arrested and charged with "impersonating a sheep hunter and
drawing knives on people"—a fitting charge against a surgeon.[21]

Once he was jailed, Duke had to be sprung. This was accomplished by
means of a gunfight, in which a good part of the population of Van Horn
bit the dust. The rest delivered Duke to Pecos, where he was brought up
before the law, the law being a local judge playing the role of Judge Roy
Bean, the hanging judge, who sentenced him—to hang. And hang Duke
did—in a harness rented from a prop department somewhere. He swung
in the breeze—a little too convincingly, Jefferson reported, since onlookers gasped as if something had gone wrong. To their collective relief, Red
was lowered to the ground and turned theatrically to the crowd.[22]

Much of the work of reintroducing bighorn sheep was done by
volunteers. Volunteers built fences and fences around the fences, dug
holes, laid pipe, installed water guzzlers to catch rainwater.[23] They did
whatever needed to be done. Duke and his cohort of friends spent about
$200,000. They were glad to. They crowed that if the state had done it,
it would have cost $2 million.[24]

There are now about 1,300 bighorns in Texas.[25]

Just as he was proud of every patient he saved, Red was proud of
every bighorn grazing the high country of West Texas. He had done
a Good Turn from his Boy Scout days that the desert bighorns would
never know a thing about. He was satisfied. "I don't know how this is
true," he said, "but they say we got as many sheep out there now as we
had in 1850."[26]

And that would gladden the hearts of Sitting Bull and Teddy Roosevelt alike.

CHAPTER 16

Living with Red Duke

Live a simple and temperate life, that you may give all your powers to your profession. Medicine is a jealous mistress; she will be satisfied with no less.
—SIR WILLIAM OSLER

Red Duke was the largely invisible center of his family's life. It revolved around his absence. As the years passed and his work grew ever more entangled with new duties and projects and more people, he spent progressively less time at home; his place at the dining table was empty night after night.

"By the time Life Flight started," Hallie says, "I was in the fourth grade and his career had consumed his life. In those years, he left for work before I got up and came home after I went to bed. I was in middle school when the TV show started. By high school, he was extremely popular, and I entered the decade of being introduced as 'Dr. Red Duke's Daughter,' as if that were my actual name."

It got worse. As fans shouting his name pursued Red and he seemed to his family more and more like a public property, Hallie began calling him Red—"because that's who he was."[1]

Red spent time with his children, but his priorities meant that he did it on his own terms: "Relating to my father meant meeting him in his world," Hallie, who has a PhD in child and family development, wrote. And the adult world was less self-consciously child-centric when the Duke children were growing up. In the 1960s and 1970s, parents were not expected to conform to their children's world so much as children were expected to conform to their parents'. Most men were less involved with their children's day-to-day lives than they are now that gender roles are less sharply divided and more mothers work. It was a rare father in the 1960s and 1970s who tied on an apron and stood at the kitchen counter making sandwiches for his children's lunchboxes.

Attention from a father was often in the nature of a treat. And that was the case even with fathers who had far fewer irons in the fire (and usually for less meritorious reasons) than Red Duke did.

Nevertheless, Red was not unaware of his children. He brought them into his life in ways that he conveniently could. Without building his life around them, he included them in the life he had. When he was going hunting, he sometimes took Hank along. Hunting and camping were adventures that not many city boys could expect to have with their fathers. Although Red might rarely be at home (something that became more conspicuous as time went on and was noticed most by the youngest child, Hallie), he was sometimes still available for church on Sundays. When he was, they attended as a family. And after church, he would sometimes take one of the children with him to the hospital as he made the rounds of his surgical patients. "We were spending time together," Hallie said, but with reservations about the suitability of the entertainment for a child. "I saw him do procedures on patients that I remember to this day—there are things you just can't unsee."

By the same token, Red would take the family to A&M football games, but, as Hallie also notes, "that was his world, too." It was one into which he could not enter anonymously, either. "To get Dr. Red Duke through a crowd of Aggie fans meant we had to turn into secret service agents and push him through the crowd with his head down, his ever-present cowboy hat hiding his face." He was often recognized anyway.

"Heaven forbid if someone saw him and shouted his name; we'd be stuck with a line of people wanting to tell him how awesome he was."

"As an adult," Hallie recalls, "spending time with him meant eating dinner at his favorite restaurant. Conversation invariably turned to his patients and the surgery he had just performed. I can't count how many times he found a paper napkin or took out one of his index cards from his shirt pocket to draw a diagram of the organs and how the procedure was done." And in restaurants fans intervened again: the children had to learn "how to watch the room. He always sat with his back to the corner or wall, but we too had to be aware if someone noticed him. At first, they would wait, but then they'd start pointing, and you knew they were talking about him. At some point, someone would build up the nerve to walk over and break through the 'private-moment-with-his-family bubble,' and that was it. Dinner had to be over, because fans would just keep coming over to talk to him."

Hallie, like the others, is quick to excuse Red's imperfections. She lays them at his father Henry's feet:

> I think the reason he was so driven is that he never felt like he was enough—not good enough, not smart enough, not hard-working enough. That was, of course, ridiculous, but he talked about it with me many times. That notion came from his father. Henry Duke was a cruel and mean man. He was brutal to Red as a child and demanded more of him than any child could give. Henry Duke was harsh and cruel to many people in the family and outside the family, but it wasn't something we talked about openly; after all, he had an image to uphold. But that meanness set Red up from an early age to feel unworthy. Red worked his whole life, up until days before he died, trying to figure out what he could do, what problem he could solve, what situation he could make better, so that he could finally prove he was "enough." He had accomplished so many amaz-ing things, improved systems and individuals' lives and trained a generation of great surgeons, but in his mind, the bar of excellence was always moving away from him. No matter how much he did or accomplished, it was never going to be enough because of the legacy his father handed him.
>
> That legacy flowed downstream. My dad's attention was on fixing great problems and saving people's lives, not on me or the family. If I needed him, or just wanted him to be around, he always had the best excuse in the world—he was saving someone's life.[2]

Betty, too, had found that excuse hard to get around. And there were others. It seemed that every spare moment away from his patients and students, Red was somewhere else. He might be hunting in distant high country, attending medical meetings or board meetings of conservation groups and charitable organizations that vied for his time, or hobnob-bing with the who's who. He did a fair amount of fundraising; he was a celebrity judge for the rodeo's annual barbeque cook-off. His televi-sion work and his star were rising fast in the eighties. But Betty at least was focused on the family. She could not make up for Red's absenteeism, but the woman who never said good-bye to her brother on the phone without saying "I love you" provided a warm, well-ordered home. She attended meticulously to the details of child-rearing, housekeeping, and the table. She supervised the children's friendships and homework and grades and hours; she kept up family ties with both Red's family and her own, and she was a close friend of Red's sister Patricia, who thought of her more as a sister than a sister-in-law.

Betty had the independence and easy self-assurance of a well-educated woman brought up with means. She was a notably good hostess, and Red, of course, was unequalled as a host. They could have thirty interns and residents over to eat on Christmas afternoon, with little fuss and no pretension. It was work, but Betty organized the children to help so that it all fell out like a well-choreographed ballet. It was for one of these parties, Rebecca wrote, that

> Mom prepared the first stacked taco I had ever seen. . . .
> Everyone would build their own plate starting with rice, then adding layers of Mom's pinto beans, taco meat, salad, Frito's narrow corn chips, and melted queso and Pace picante sauce on top. Some years Dad oversaw the process for making the frozen margaritas and a frozen drink that was made from fruit juices and wine. I still have a copy of "his" margarita recipe handwritten on an old index card and remember him meticulously reciting instructions for mixing together cans of frozen fruit juice with tequila or wine as if we were making a rare beverage that we were quite privileged to know the special recipe for. Even making simple syrup for the margaritas became a chemistry lesson with dad reciting step-by-step instructions, adding in scientific lessons about the properties of sugar and water. All that we learned was typically linked to a patient he was treating to complete the teaching moment at hand.
>
> The ritual started in large vats the day before, which were put in the upright freezer out in the laundry room. I enjoyed stirring the mix at regular intervals to keep the freezing crystals small and smooth for drinking. In hindsight that was long before anyone had ever dreamed of having a frozen drink machine at home. It felt as if we were conjuring up quite a

bohemian concoction for this party, and I was particularly intrigued to witness both my parents diverting from their strict Southern Baptist background for the events of the day.

Dad would play his latest favorite record for each new arrival at the party. Some records were country music favorites, but he also loved the recordings of some funny old-timers spinning yarns about chasing 'coons up trees and other antics, each story having a wry moral lesson at the end. He would put on a record and gather a few folks to listen. If he thought your attention was waning he'd point at the record player and say in a loud voice, "Now listen to this!" as he did not want you to miss the point of the song's sermon.

Dad's day was not over until he had made a trip to the hospital. He often took food to the interns, nurses, and certain patients who were not lucky enough to go home for holidays. After the festivities at home were over, leftovers from any family feast would be packed up and delivered to the hospital. I went with him on many occasions and we walked many miles down the corridors of Hermann Hospital. Here he would show me around his world with a twinkle in his eye while he delivered food as if he was one of Santa's elves. As he hugged, teased, and talked with folks, it was easy to see how good they felt that he had not forgotten them. It was not hard to see that this was where he felt at home.[3]

As the margaritas demonstrate, Red could whip the ordinary into the wonderful. He was a Rumpelstiltskin, spinning straw into gold:

Dad took small things and made them seem epic. I remember how both my parents, especially my dad, would discover new foods and drinks and then incorporate them into our family story. When we moved to New York, they found a small family-run restaurant in Little Italy that served a fettuccini dish that they loved. They became friendly with the owner and asked how to make it. Soon the fettuccini and the story about the people who made it was a family standard. Dad told and retold that story until it took on a life of its own. I don't remember the details anymore, but that fettuccini still tastes extra special when I make it.

The enthusiasm and exactitude with which Dad examined and consumed life was rigorous and oftentimes unforgiving, but it is also one of the gifts I received from him. I do not know what it means to feel bored and cannot imagine what life is like without having a passionate interest in many things.[4]

Of all the children, Sara is perhaps most reminiscent of her father. She has a bit of his look, his coloring, a touch of his manner. Red introduced her on my first breakfast visit to her home. "God did give me a blessing in her, and she is tough. She is driven. She got a PhD in plant physiology. She is a scientist at heart. She thinks like a scientist. She had a degree in math from A&M, and then after she got her PhD she got a master's in statistics, and that is an interesting thing."[5] When he was ill, it was to Sara that Red first turned. He convalesced for nearly eight months under her care in her College Station home with her family. While she shares her siblings' childhood memories of her father—spending Christmas Day with his students and colleagues, following him around the hospital—she also has another perspective on living with Red. When he was weak and debilitated after his surgery, Sara was the daughter who took care of him and experienced a reversal of roles with him, providing the immediate help he needed.

As a child Sara had adored her father. Caring for him when he was old and ill made her feel a new closeness to him. That feeling was reciprocated, and it was a new bond between them. Sara was his spokesperson when he received awards or attended events, and she needed no script to tell everyone in attendance about his love of medicine and of people. Her husband, Charles, recalls how much he learned from Red during those months when they shared a roof. "I used to jump to conclusions about people and judge people without knowing them," Charles says. "Red cured me of that. He always had another perspective—that we should get to know people, not judge them on the surface. He had this sensitivity to others and their feelings that would make this world a better place if we all approached life like Red. It just didn't matter to him if you were president of the United States or some poor soul sleeping under a bridge—you mattered to Red."[6]

Ask Sara to summarize her father in a word and you will hear about his courage in the end. "He dealt with so much pain and discomfort without complaint. At times he just felt like crap, but you'd never know it. He put others around him first and minimized his own problems. That courage I will live with and never forget nor cease to admire."[7]

The girls did not present Red and Betty with a great many occasions to dispense discipline as they were growing up, but Hank was another matter entirely. Betty for the most part left disciplining Hank to Red, who, Hank reports, "was not a great authoritarian, because he just wasn't home that much. However, I can remember being awakened many a time late at night when he returned from the hospital, to catch his wrath for something I had done during the day that he felt merited a good whipping. He improved on his father's behavior, but when it came to discipline, I have to say the apple didn't fall far from the tree."[8]

One instance of coming to grief that Hank especially remembers was the day in 1972 when he and his father were leaving Afghanistan to return to the States. The plane was waiting for them, but Hank, in a fit of teenage rebellion, was not cooperating. "I didn't want to go. Mom and my sisters had already departed several days earlier, and Dad and I were to fly back when he finished up his hospital business. I ran away to a friend's house and hid. I wanted to stay. Dad had to comb the streets of Jalalabad to find me, and he did. I can tell you he wasn't too happy about that stunt. It was one of my first and boldest outright rebellions."[9] It would not be the last. Hank was full of the devil.

• • •

In 1982 Red Duke started the year with a letter to his parents that provided a snapshot of Christmas Day in the Duke household. The children were all there, he wrote; multiple things were going on at once and everybody pitched in to help; the new grandbaby, "Grunt," was a neophyte this Christmas but could be counted on to have expertise in the celebration by the next one; there was food, conversation, music, storytelling, and general revelry; by afternoon there were thirty-five guests to join in it all; and the hit of the day, the highlight of the celebration, was the electric train that Helen and Hank had sent. The package had guarded its secrets so well that everyone had imagined the contents to be a framed picture. They had set the track up on the oak table and everyone had admired it extravagantly in every detail, right down to the perfection with which it fit into its space. There was a little family news about tonsils and a hunting trip with Hank and good performances at school, and an obscure conclusion: "I wish we could have been with you Christmas, but I understand, and think you did the best thing. Thank you again for your kindness." The closing was "Sincerely" (January 6, 1982).

Something was obviously afoot. Perhaps the penultimate sentence refers to the serpent in the idyllic picture Red has just painted of the Duke family Christmas. Within eight months, Red and Betty would be separated. In 1984 they would be divorced.

"Red left the house in the fall of 1982 to move into an apartment and to file for a divorce," Betty said. "I went to the Dukes' for Thanksgiving because I felt more accepted there. My family did not support the divorce. They just could not see it, did not want it, and I did. I can say that despite their feelings about divorce, I did feel loved and supported by my family through it all."[10]

Red and Betty had long been drifting. He was a television personality, a surgeon and a professor of surgery, and a public person who travelled in high circles and had little time left for a home life. Betty, who had given up her own teaching career and raised four children on the go from Texas to Afghanistan, was tired, admittedly depressed, and little interested in fancy events studded with celebrities. Since Red loved to hobnob and Betty did not, he hobnobbed and she stayed at home and dreamed about a quiet life in the country like the one she had known in her girlhood. She was an independent woman at heart, and Red was on the fast track to somewhere else. They tried counseling. It didn't work.

Hank had noticed that his parents were drifting apart several years before his father moved out. Hallie, the youngest, was just fifteen. While Red had not been around the house for daily activities in many years, she recalls, the separation and eventual divorce made his absence very real, and she felt it deeply. But, painful as it was, she says, it also ended up being a catalyst for healing, because it was honest. There was now no mistaking, no pretense about what came first for her father. It was medicine.

Red, not without pain himself, turned to his medical family. Eventually—for the last twenty years of his life—he would literally live in the hospital around the clock, making time when he could to see the children and celebrate holidays with the family.

When Betty recalls the early days of their marriage, before the children came along and when responsibilities were few and fame had not yet swallowed them, what stands out to her is that they shared power in the relationship. "We were equals then," she says, "and I had a say in everything we did together."

If you asked Red and Betty Duke for a favorite memory from the past, they would independently tell you about their 1957 road trip to Alaska. It was a trip they planned together to celebrate the successful completion of Red's first year of medical school. They would meet new people and see gorgeous sights—snow-covered mountains and crystal-blue glaciers that no picture in any magazine could duplicate. It was a brief, idyllic interlude for the young couple, before different interests and different demands set them on diverging paths. It was a dream-chasing time.

Red had long been looking for a job in Alaska, but nothing had turned up, so the couple bought a Ford ranch wagon and hit the road. The idea was to support themselves by working as they traveled. They followed the old, partly unpaved Alaskan highway, a 1,500-mile road constructed during World War II and connecting the United States to Alaska across Canada. The road was pitted with holes and strewn with rocks "too big to be called gravel," to which they lost a headlight, and they drove into a rainstorm that followed them for the next five hundred miles over barely passable wooden bridges and washouts. They were exquisitely happy, traveling snugly together through a wet, threatening wilderness at twenty-five and thirty miles an hour—which was as fast as the combination of road and weather would permit.

They looked forward to Anchorage, which promised a bath. "I do not think that we will ever live up here," Red pronounced. "I do not think that I could ever be very efficient because there are too many lakes that need to be relieved of their overstocked fish population and there are too many valleys that have not been seen"[11] (July 1, 1957). The mountains were immensely tall and lay under blankets of snow.

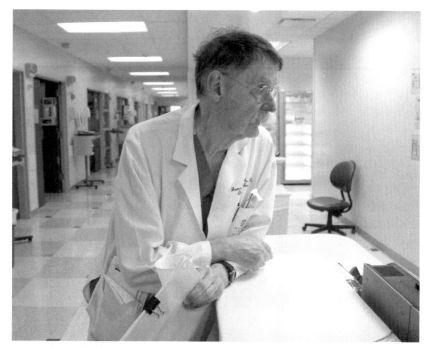

Red on the wards of Memorial Hermann Hospital–Texas Medical Center, his pockets full of index cards and notes. Visiting patients, rushing to surgery, he knew no night or day. Courtesy of Dwight C. Andrews.

They drove into a job in Mountain View, just outside Anchorage. There Red was hired by the Bureau of Land Management to fight fires, "but they figured with all those degrees I had I could probably make up the packs to drop those fire fighters."[12] For accommodations, they found a church whose pastor would put them up at his home for the reasonable price of a few odd jobs and leading some prayer groups. "This is certainly an answer to prayer," Red wrote home, "for I am working within three miles of the church and the pastor's home where we are presently staying. I am not too crazy about the work, but for the present it is a job and pays more money than I have ever made. They pay $2.78/hour and for every 8 hours work I get a credit of 9 hours for the subsistence that I am not receiving as do the fire fighters in the bush" (July 14, 1957).

Their Alaskan adventure filled the entire summer of 1957. At the end of the summer Red sold the car to the pastor and they flew home,

Red to rejoin his classmates at medical school and Betty to return to teaching.

Now, three decades later, Red was single again—or, more accurately, married to medicine. His life was centered on it. He would have other loves in his life, even remarry for five years, but his deepest love would always be for medicine. It always won out in the end.

Divorce did not change Red's life very much, because he hadn't been living a domestic life anyway. He hadn't gone home for dinner with any regularity before the divorce, so when he still didn't, it made little difference other than that now the place he didn't go home to was an apartment instead of the house. Before, he had run into his children occasionally—mainly Hallie, because she was the one still at home. Now when he saw them it was by design, but he was too deeply into his own occupations to do much designing.

But even though the divide between himself and his family had been established long before, the officialness of divorce, which had struck Hallie as cleansing in its honesty, must have stricken Red with a sense of his isolation. In spite of the hospital and the swarms of his acquaintance there, in spite of the consolations of the wilderness and his hunting buddies, in spite of the familiar and collegial chattering and gabbling of professional societies, and in spite of the television cameras and the care and tending of his celebrity, Red had to be alone sometimes, and to face the fact that the fundamental relationship in his life was gone. He must have had to face that fact in a way that he did not have to face it before the divorce. He was free, but he was unmoored.

Except by medicine.

CHAPTER 17

Second Marriages

A year after the divorce, Red Duke was on his way back to Houston from a medical conference in San Antonio when by chance he took a seat in the front of the plane for the one-hour flight and found himself directly across the aisle from an attractive woman dressed in full western wear. She was Pamela Ann Martens, a native Houstonian and interior decorator, who had been in Kerrville that week, drawing up design plans for a client's new ranch house. She had been in a hurry as she left for the plane straight from the ranch and hadn't had time to change. She felt a little self-conscious about her cowboy boots and western garb on the plane, but it was a short hop home. She noticed that the tall man who had loped down the aisle to the seat across from her was wearing boots and jeans and a cowboy hat. "Well, I'm dressed fine," she thought.

> And I'm sitting in my seat, and he sits in the seat directly across from me, in the other aisle seat. And I don't think anything of it. I sit down and I pull the in-flight magazine right in front of me. And there's a picture of this doctor on the front with the scrub hat and his scrubs on. And I look at that picture, look over at him, and I think, "Nah, that isn't him." And then the guy—I start reading the article, and then he speaks to me in that loud voice, because you can't hear and they started the engine. And I look over at him, and I hold up this thing, and I point at it. Now I've got to believe it's him. And I go, "This you?" And he goes, "Yeah."
>
> Anyway, we fly to Houston, I stand up, and he takes my luggage, my hanging bag, out of my hand. He says, "Here, I'll carry this, young lady." And we go walking to the garage, and we end up sitting down there on one of those curbs in the garage and just talking. And he says, "Well, let's go have a dinner. Do you like fish?" And I'm like, "Yeah, I love fish. I

predominantly eat seafood." He said, "Well, we'll just go split a fish." And I was like, "Okay."

So he came to pick me up . . . in a pickup truck. And at that point, the pickup truck had . . . kind of like a felt liner, I guess. It was at the top of it and had fallen down, and there was like fabric that rested on the top of my head. "Have you ever thought of maybe getting this fixed before it falls down into your eyes or something, or getting a new truck?" "Oh, hell, no, baby. I got a lot more time on this truck." Anyway, we went and split a fish, and were together ever after.[1]

It was this chance encounter that led to Red's second marriage. Pam, single like Red, had also been married before. She was twenty years younger than Red, and younger by the same amount than her previous husband, Kenneth Schnitzer. Schnitzer was a prominent and often colorful developer of major Houston properties, including Greenway Plaza, Hudson on Memorial, and the Houston Summit, which in later years was the home of Joel Osteen's Lakewood Church. As an interior

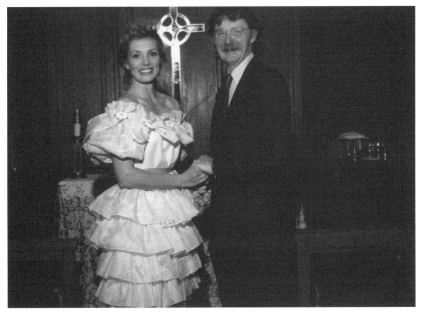

Pam and Red Duke's wedding day, Palmer Episcopal Church, Houston 1989.

decorator, Pam had had a hand in all these projects. And she was known for her work on the Houston charity circuit.

After several years of dating, Red and Pam were married in 1989 at Palmer Episcopal Church, right across the street from Hermann Hospital. They exchanged vows in a small, private ceremony.

They were a couple in steady demand for appearances at the competing fundraising events that fill the city's hotel ballrooms every weekend. Red, who during his first marriage had not found time to go home to dinner, now managed to don black ties and cummerbunds and to dazzle and be dazzled by Houston society. Houston, the fourth largest city in the country, is known for its philanthropy, and Red and Pam helped raise untold monies for good causes. Among their favorite events was the annual Houston Livestock and Rodeo, perhaps the signature event of the year, which yields millions of dollars for student scholarships and other good causes. Here the couple were active on committees and as guests, more than once riding in the famed Salt Grass Trail Ride's Wagon 7.

Chili cook-offs were favorite affairs of Red's. He loved the cold weather, the chili, the beer, and the bourbon—these were much closer to his taste than fancy ballrooms and formal dress codes. (When a group from the hospital would duck out at night to eat nearby, a ritual question was, "What's the dress code?" The ritual answer was, "Green," meaning, we can go in scrubs, which made everyone happy, especially Red.[2]) When Red and Pam were not in Houston consorting with the local beau monde, they might be found in Austin on Willie Nelson's bus. Red more than once helped out at Farm Aid and other Willie Nelson charity concerts, offering up his medical expertise. "Big crowds, a hot sun, and alcohol are a prescription for calamity," he would preach. His practiced ability to plan and deliver medical logistics for these immense events was welcome, and it added to the growing list of country and rock artists he came to know over the years.

But an event in 1990, not long after he and Pam were married, stands out as both memorable and prophetic. They were in Los Angeles for a medical conference and were staying at one of Pam's favorite hotels, L'Ermitage, "which for Red was a push." (Red preferred cheaper lodgings.) They were going out for dinner. "So we go push the button for the elevator. The elevator door opens. It's Willie and Waylon, it's Kris, and it's Johnny Cash, standing right in front of us."

Willie Nelson, Waylon Jennings, Kris Kristofferson, and Johnny Cash had formed the supergroup the Highwaymen in 1985. They sang a unique brand of country music—outlaw country—that made their first collaborative album a major hit and defined a new genre. The title song, "Highwaymen," landed at the top of country charts that year. Now the four country icons were back in town to record a second Highwaymen album.

After some conversation, "They go, 'Hey, Red. You and Pam want to come watch us record tomorrow? We're doing the *Highwaymen 2*. Come on over.' And Red goes, 'Well, I've got to go to this meeting. But Pam can go with you.'"

The next day Pam was in a recording studio and Red was at his American College of Surgeons conference. Nothing would have pleased

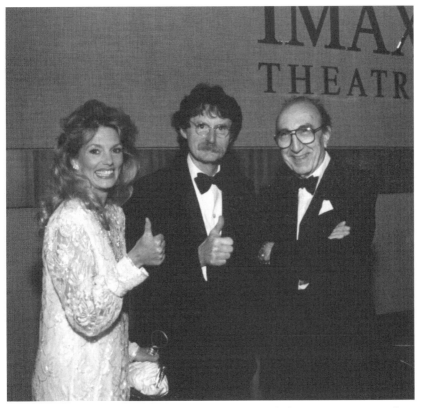

Red and Pam with Michael DeBakey at a Houston event in the late 1980s. Courtesy of Pam Duke.

him better than to watch musical history being made (*Highwaymen 2*, like the first album, was a hit, and it was nominated for a Grammy that year). Yet Red was deep into the business of medicine. When he wasn't at the hospital, he was keeping up with the latest buzz at conferences, fraternizing with fellow surgeons, and comparing medical notes. Meanwhile, across town, Pam tapped her boots to the musical notes of the Highwaymen. Even hobnobbing now was taking a back seat to medicine. It was a formula not exactly for disaster, as it worked out, but certainly for dissolution.

Five years after Red and Pam married, they agreed amicably to divorce. Pam felt that she had already conquered Houston—had decorated everything in it that she wanted to decorate and had worked for every charitable cause in town—and that it was time to move on. Moreover, she said, "I really, truly knew that I wanted to go live in Kerrville, which my grandparents had moved to in '47. And I had a house there. . . . It was partially me, but the other thing was with Red; he had pretty much—he was living and sleeping in the hospital more than he was at home." And his reasons were as always righteous; they were unimpeachable; they could not even be decently argued with. He was saving lives. Pam recounts her unsuccessful attempts to make plans with her husband:

> "Oh, I really want to go to the whatever tonight. Can we go?"
> "Sure, we can go." And then the pager would go off, and it would be, "Oh, I'm sorry. So-and-so just came in, and they're bleeding out. I've got to go."
> And it's like, "Okay."
> Because you can't argue with a bleeding pager.

Red's marriage to Pam was an important phase in his life, and the friendship that grew out of it survived the marriage. They were divorced in 1994, for the same reasons for which he had been divorced in 1984. But Red never cast a love or a friendship casually aside. Several years later, he cheerfully agreed to meet his former wife and her new fiancé, Greg, in the Turks and Caicos Islands (southeast of the Bahamas) to read scripture for their wedding. Red and Greg became fast friends and hunting buddies—among other places, they hunted together in the mountains of Alaska. They called themselves "husbands-in-law." Eventually, Pam said, "they were going on hunting trips and meeting at hunting shows without me."

It would be Red's last attempt at marriage. Working around the clock in the hospital, he had his medical family. Medicine would hold him close to the hospital for the rest of his life.

One former medical colleague, Celeste Sheppard, recalls the day some months after his divorce from Pam that a once-again single Red Duke asked her if she wanted to have a cup of coffee. They became frequent dinner partners over the next two years while she worked at Hermann Hospital and the medical school. "I would have married that girl if she had been a few years older," he once told me.[3] She was thirty; he was sixty-five. "We almost never talked about it," she said, "but that's a thirty-five-year-sized elephant in the room."[4]

At the time Red was living with one foot in a grim apartment on Braeswood, jammed with taxidermy and stacked with rugs from Afghanistan, and the other in "an old call room in his office at the hospital." He much preferred the call room, Celeste thought. "I remember he used to say it was the best thing ever. He said, 'When my second foot hits the ground, my commute is over.' Just a very Red thing to say."[5]

Red was packing a handgun in those days. "As I understand it," Celeste says, "the brother of one of Red's trauma patients, who died despite the trauma team's efforts, was rumored to be making threats against Red's life among his friends and family. . . . I think someone who heard this guy talking (I think it was a family member) sent a letter to Red about the threat." Thus,

> before the police put a detail person on him, Red started carrying Elizabeth, who was a 9 mm. It was a big gun and he would carry it in the back of his waistband when outside the hospital and medical school. At that time we were going to dinner pretty much every night. . . . It was just kind of funny because people could sometimes see it.
>
>   At this time, his completely predictable uniform was his boots, jeans, a tailored handmade shirt, and a blue blazer. He wore that everywhere. But sometimes his jacket would get caught up on the handle of the gun so you could see it. So here

is the man who is sort of famous for, you know, accidents don't just happen, and he has a handgun stuck in his belt. . . . And the restaurateurs kind of got used to it—they'd stare at the gun handle and ask, "Everything okay, Dr. Duke?" Red would pull the jacket over. "Yes, yes, everything is fine."[6]

After about six months the police escort was dropped. Red was not entirely happy about that, because he believed in the malevolence of his former patient's brother, but Celeste saw that it gave him one more excuse to keep living in the hospital. The real reason was more that it was a clean, well-lighted place. The break with Pam had been amiable enough, but it had left Red wounded and lonelier than he would admit:

> He had . . . moved into the musty, dark apartment that was indeed chockablock with his treasures and probably hundreds of plaques and mementoes—but there was little furniture and the kitchen was cramped and neglected. He mostly kept to-go containers in the fridge, some good bourbon and tequila on the countertop, and, of course, a coffeemaker. This really was more of a campsite than a home. The bedroom was like a cave—he preferred to sleep in pitch blackness and had hung a TAMU blanket over the window to keep out any stray light. There was a television in the bedroom but he used it exclusively to play tapes of Willie Nelson or Kris Kristofferson or Roger Miller concerts, Western movies, National Geographic shows about Alaska, or the documentary about his west Texas bighorn sheep program. What I remember best was watching videos of outtakes from his UT-TV segment. We would watch those outtake tapes, maybe a little giddy from the tequila, and laugh until gasping for air at the hilarious bloopers.[7]

In time Red let the apartment go and replaced it with two storage units near the Texas Medical Center. These he filled with a lifetime collection of memorabilia, including several well-aged boxes of yellowed letters that would form the framework of much of this book. From the middle of 1995, the hospital was his home. Celeste describes his lifestyle there as minimalist. "He had three pairs of socks. He had sort of one to wear, one to wash, and one folded up ready to go. Two or three pairs of shorts, and he would wash them in the sink. He called it 'living like a coyote' and he kind of liked it."[8]

His calendar was filled, but now with hunting and conservation work, rather than galas and high society. It was the hospital he came home to, Celeste writes:

> In the post-Pam (and post-Celeste) periods, I really think he came even more deeply to regard the Life Flight team as his family. I think he liked living in the hospital because of the ready access to the Life Flight office, staffed 24/7 with people who shared his mission passionately and who risked their lives for the program he founded and nurtured. He would wander up there in the middle of the night to have a cup of coffee with the dispatchers. He was in charge of writing the surgery call schedule and nearly always put himself on call on holidays. This was interpreted as generosity to his colleagues with families—but I think it was a way to fill his loneliness and spend time with the people who had become de facto his family. . . . He filled his time with doctoring—which was the central manifestation of his nurturing instinct [and his] identity.[9]

Betty went to work after the divorce. "Hallie had just graduated from high school," she said, "and I prayed to God, 'What am I going to do now? Hallie's gone.'" So she found a job. "I was on the board for the Odyssey House, a nonprofit residential treatment program to help adolescents with alcohol and chemical abuse problems. We had hired a man who [then stole] from us, using our credit card. . . . We fired that man, and I said, 'Oh, I can do that job. He was dishonest and inept. I am ept and honest.'" Betty was named executive director and helped raise the money to get the program started in Houston.[10]

Having decamped to the Presbyterian church (much to her mother's displeasure), Betty met Pete Kent, a widower, in a Presbyterian singles class. "They had a big singles ministry. Pete and I were at the dance where you switch partners throughout. . . . He and I partnered and that was the beginning of our relationship and marriage."[11]

They married in 1990. At sixty-three, Pete was two years Betty's senior. He was a widower whose first wife had left him with two adopted children, who were now both grown. And so Betty and Pete found each other and danced. It was about the time they both retired. "I had bought an early Texas farmhouse built in 1870 on nine acres, just before Red and I were divorced," Betty said. This was what they would call the New Ulm Farm. New Ulm is a small town located between Brenham and Columbus. "I bought it *feme sole*. I didn't know that term until then, and I've heard it very seldom since. . . . I just fell in love with that house. I restored it and put my heart and soul into it. I had for years been buying and selling antiques, and I had made quite a collection of early Texas furniture." So she already had exactly what the house needed.

Both Kents developed an interest in gourds. Although gourds have been decorated for centuries as a folk craft, they have lately attracted attention even in legitimate arts communities. Betty and Pete began growing gourds, which is an art in itself, and then shaping them into bowls, lamp bases, and other functional objects. Betty stained them; Pete cut them. He could carve waves and intricate designs and make lids that fit perfectly. He was very creative and even designed innovative cutting tools. Together the pair taught classes in growing gourds and in techniques for shaping and cutting them. Pete's techniques and tools were always part of teaching demonstrations at the arts fairs they attended. They both loved traveling to the shows.

A leisurely country life in an old Texas farmhouse that she loved, traveling to art and craft and antique shows, and marriage to an easygoing, companionable man who had time to dance with her, was everything that Betty wanted. The Austin County home provided a congenial place for the children and grandchildren of both families to gather at Thanksgiving and Easter. "And Red would often come to the dinner to be with us," Betty says:

> He and Pete got along very well. In fact, when Hallie got married in 2000 . . . he was there to give [her] away for her wedding.
>
> I was seated on the front row and then they brought Pete down to sit beside me. Red walked Hallie down the aisle, and then he came and turned around and sat on the other side of me. I could hardly maintain decorum thinking, "I'm sitting

here between two husbands." And then when they walked
us out of the service, the ushers came to get me and both Red
and Pete got up behind me, and the three of us walked out
together. I'm sure I controlled myself but I was giggling on the
inside.[12]

When Pete died in 2013, Red was there with family and friends to help
Betty scatter his ashes at the New Ulm farm. Although Red's love life
was messy at times, and when his marriages ended, he was not happy,
what he looked for and found was friendship rather than bitterness in
the rubble. "I'm not perfect," he was almost too quick to say, and he was
right. One of his imperfections was that balancing family life and medicine was a skill he would never master.

But when all that was left was medicine, he found a family in that.

CHAPTER 18
Working with Red Duke

The good physician treats the disease,
  the great physician treats the patient who has the disease
—Sir William Osler

In many ways Red Duke's hospital patients, his professional colleagues, and the thousands of students who hung on his words in the lecture hall and followed him on patient rounds during his fifty-four years in medicine were his family as much as the family at home was. Some might say that in later years they were his primary family. He was in constant motion as he hurried between surgeries, lecture halls, and television shoots. He was everywhere, congenial and gregarious, making and remaking human connections wherever he turned. And those who worked near him, the doctors, nurses, students, and TV crews, all have favorite stories to tell.

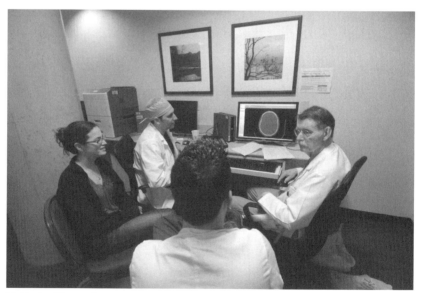

Red in teaching mode.

"Hi, Sweetie!" and "Hey, Bud!" rang out in Hermann's busy corridors as Red greeted friends and stranger alike in his Texas twang. Assigning nicknames to his colleagues was a famous Duke practice. I overheard one surgeon telling several others that Red had always called him "Hoss." He looked very pleased. Then, after a pause, he added, "But I think I was one of two hundred Hosses." Richard Andrassy, chairman of the medical school's surgery department, was "Bugger" and proud of it, indicating that political correctness and adjustments for rank were not part of Red's big picture.

Dukeisms coined (or pirated) by Red were another trademark that endeared him to his public. When asked where they came from, he shrugged and said, "I don't know. Some I make up. Some I just steal outright."

Red's mentor in medical school, Don Seldin, was memorably aphoristic when he taught. Red carried the practice further, creating one-liners (some shamelessly pilfered from Seldin himself) indelible enough that every student would take away a trove of them. Most, when queried, can readily recall a prized Dukeism even decades later. Here are some favorites:

He's two or three bubbles off plumb.

Any day above ground is a good day.

He's as crazy as a two-pecker owl.

Stay in the high grass and don't raise your head in the same place twice.

Don't punch a skunk.

You only get into the ICU two ways . . . by being stupid or being with stupid.

It ain't the fall that's so bad; it's the sudden stop that hurts.

To a student about to make a mistake:

Son, you sure you want to saddle that horse?

To an overzealous medical student who was asked for more suture during surgery:

Honey, we're not trying to build a trotline.

To surgical colleague Jim Bertz's wife, who marveled to Red that everybody at the hospital adored him:

If you love them a lot, they will like you a little.

To a Life Flight pilot whose reflexes were a little slower than Red's:

Are you going to shut this lawnmower down?

A year after Red died, Memorial Hermann honored him and the anniversary of Life Flight with an exhibit in the hospital's Rick Smith Gallery. It included photographs, memorabilia, and stories written by Red's colleagues. Those stories provide snapshots of what working with Red was like.[1]

Cissy Rivers, a longtime veteran of the hospital's food services, remembers her first hug with Dr. Duke:

> I was working the cash register at Café Hermann one evening after suffering an injury to my arm. I had been in excruciating pain for two weeks and my doctor hadn't yet figured out what was wrong, so he put me in a brace. Dr. Duke came to my register to pay for his food when he noticed me holding my swollen arm. He told me, "Take that darn thing off your arm." Within seconds, he told me I had gout and said I needed to go back to the doctor for an X-ray. Sure enough, Dr. Duke was right.
>
> The next week he stopped by my register to check on me. I was already feeling a hundred times better than the week before. But when I told him what medicine my doctor had prescribed, Dr. Duke looked just as annoyed as the day he told me to take off my brace. He asked me for the doctor's phone number so he could call and get me the right prescription. And he did. . . . The next time he came to the café to check on me, I asked if I could give him a hug. I hugged that man with all the

love and gratitude in my heart—just the hugs my granny used to give me—and I felt all the muscles and bones in his body relax. He came back the next evening for another hug and every day after that for the next five years.[2]

As an ordained minister, Red more than a few times performed wedding ceremonies for colleagues. Billy Gill and Michelle McNutt, fellow trauma surgeons, asked Red to marry them in their backyard. Recalls Gill, "While the ceremony was going on, his dog Jake was playing in the pool. As we were exchanging our vows and holding hands, Jake came up and shook that pool water all over us. For some, I imagine that would have been a disaster, but for us, it was a wonderful thing. . . . When our twins were born, we named our son James after Dr. Duke. Hopefully our son also inherited a piece of Dr. Duke's generous soul."[3]

Joseph Love had completed his surgical residency when he was first interviewed by Red, who conducted the interview at lunch. Love, still on active duty with the air force, had just returned from Afghanistan. "I was given orders from the US Air Force to be stationed in either Pittsburgh or Houston. The goal was to create a platform in a busy civilian hospital to maintain readiness for deployment. Houston was a natural fit. Red and I shared stories about the military and Afghanistan and our relationship grew from there. He was a genuine person, never truly comfortable with being 'famous' or recognizable."[4]

Love still recalls that interview near the Texas Medical Center. Red pulled his beaten up old truck into the parking lot of a busy Mexican restaurant and stopped, while waving cars around him.

If it had been me driving, I probably would have gotten my truck keyed. But because it was Dr. Duke, people just drove around us and waved. Inside the restaurant Red greeted everyone in the kitchen before grabbing a takeout box and filling it with tomatoes and onions from the salad bar. He kept talking and warned me that I might think some of what he said was offensive, but that he was always going to tell me how it is. That was one of the things I loved about him. He wasn't interested in going out of his way to make you feel comfortable with who he was.

He was also a pivotal person in my children's lives. . . . My kids would see him at parties, gatherings, and dedications, and I would make sure they spent time and talked with him. When he was ill they wanted to visit him when they could after school. On several occasions they had their class at school draw prayer cards, which I brought to him. He read each one and even had his daughter Sara put together a folder for the cards so he could look them over as he wanted to. Kids and education were extremely important to him, and as he aged, "kids" became a loose term to include older ones, like me.[5]

After Red's death, Love was named medical director of Life Flight. "I may have his old title," he said, "but I'll never fill his shoes. He was one of a kind."

One attribute that more than a few veteran physicians working with Red on the hospital side remember was his ability to recall patient numbers. Some swear that even years after he had seen a patient, Red could recall her number from the charts at a moment's notice. But while knowing the patient's number for the chart was convenient, knowing her name for her care was imperative. Many a young doctor who referred to a patient by a number in front of Red was quickly silenced and ordered back to the patient's bedside to return with a name. "We're treating a person, not a disease. Never forget that," he would insist. It was a lesson no student escaped.

Giuseppe Colasurdo, president of UTHealth, remembers that even in Red's last days, students were never far from his mind. He asked the president to promise continued support for the school's scholarship programs. In their last conversation, Colasurdo recalls that Red said, "Never forget, those students need all the help they can get."[6] Even in his eighties, Red could remember what it felt like to be a cash-strapped student who had to calculate the price of gas into his decision whether to go home for a weekend. And for many students it was much worse. For many it was a case of whether they could afford their degrees at all. Red never lost the power to empathize.

Logan Rutherford, a Memorial-Hermann hospital chaplain, had much in common with Red (including admiration for Albert Schweitzer). Rutherford likes to tell the story of Red's sympathy for the

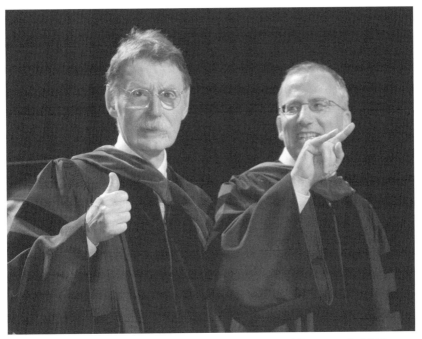

Dr. Red Duke and UTHealth President Dr. Giuseppe Colasurdo, following Red's 2008 medical school commencement address. Courtesy of Dwight C. Andrews.

trauma nurses. "Over the years, I witnessed profound examples of service from Dr. Duke on a daily basis—one in particular stays with many of us to this day. He knew how hard the nurses in the Shock Trauma ICU worked and knew they did not have the ability to go farther than their staff lounge to eat lunch. So every day Dr. Duke would collect the leftover food from the physician dining room and wheel it to the break room for the staff to eat instead of letting it go to waste."[7]

Perhaps no one in the hospital knew Red better than Tom Flanagan. Flanagan began his career as a nurse and transitioned to become a flight nurse with Life Flight. In time he was promoted to vice-president and chief operating officer for the entire hospital.

Flanagan loved Red Duke. He knew him first as the doctor on television. Consequently, when he interviewed with Red for the Air Ambulance service, he was nervous and self-conscious. But Duke set him at ease. The interview turned to Alaska and sheep hunting. "There's not much I know about Alaska," Flanagan said, "and there's certainly not much I know about hunting sheep. But for some reason he took a chance on me, and that began a thirty-year relationship. More than professional, he was my mentor, he was a colleague, and at the end of the day he was really a father to me."

Red counseled Tom through rough patches:

> Now, I will tell you there were discussions that were frank and honest, requiring a little more humility for me, which I value today. And every time I walked out of a discussion—personal, professional, didn't matter—I walked away with a little bit more wisdom, a little bit more knowledge, and I always walked away thinking I was right on top of the world. That was one of the many, many talents . . . Dr. Duke had. There wasn't a person in this organization that he wouldn't walk by and stop and recognize, say hello, spend time [with], ask how they were, how was their family. He was a stranger to none.[8]

And then there are the patients, an endless line of patients and family members all of whom have a story to tell and an inner prompting to thank Red Duke. Here is just one. Until the day he died, James Mitchell remembered the night his only son was in an automobile crash and underwent severe trauma to his face. His wife retells her late husband's story, one typical of countless tributes from patients and family members Red treated over the years.

> James . . . had just talked to our son's surgeon, who left him to ponder . . . [the] pain and long recovery ahead. My husband stepped outside into the hall. Numerous physicians hurried down that busy corridor, but one stopped and looked him in the eye. It was Red Duke, who saw the tears on his face and slowed to his side. "You OK? What can I do for you? Want me to go check on your son and give you a report?" James was not only shocked to recognize Red Duke; he was impressed that perhaps the busiest doctor in the whole place was the one to volunteer his time for a total stranger. James remarked later that he would never forget the compassion and care he felt at that moment. Our son recovered and is doing fine. In a way,

my husband recalled, he got a good dose of medicine himself that night. He had met Red Duke and witnessed a kindness and compassion that you just don't see every day.[9]

To the thousands of medical students he taught over the years, Red was a role model for professionalism and setting priorities—specifically, putting the patient first. One doctor, a second-year medical student at the time, remembers walking by Red with a bandage on her finger from a kitchen mishap the day before. "It was a Monday morning and Red Duke spotted me in that crowded hall and asked about the bandage. Within minutes he was cleaning my cut and adding a couple of stitches in a nearby clinical station before sending me on my way with a wink and a smile. He was out there in the hall between surgeries cheering his students on and ready at a moment's notice to [fill] any need he might spot. I knew that very day that was the kind of doctor I wanted to be."

Jim Bertz, a maxillofacial surgeon with both medical and dental degrees, remembers Red Duke as far back as his medical-school days in Dallas. Bertz, now retired and living in Scottsdale, Arizona, is still volunteering his surgical talents for patients around the world. He remembers the first time he met Red Duke:

It was 1963, and he was the first guy I met when I arrived at UT Southwestern. I was looking for the OMFS Clinic and he walked by. He was busy, but when I asked for help, he said, "Come on, I'll show you." I am sure that was the last thing he wanted to do, but in the Red Duke tradition, he was helping poor, lost souls. I actually remember what he was wearing. He had a blue button-down shirt, khaki pants, a tie and those horn-rim glasses with short hair. When The Creator sent his molds to make mankind, he sent one apart from all others, the one that made Red Duke. He has no twin.[10]

In the late 1970s Bertz found himself in Peshawar, Pakistan, at the Afghan Surgical Hospital for Refugees.

I was caring for Afghans wounded in their battle with the Russians. Dr. Rabani was the chief of surgery there at the time, and I asked him where he had trained, and he said,

"Jalalabad." Of course I asked him if he knew the name Red
Duke, and to my surprise, tears came to his eyes. He asked,
"You know Red Duke? He trained me." He asked me to bring
Dr. Duke on our next trip and because of [our connection to]
Dr. Duke, we all were given bodyguards from that moment on.
Dr. Duke's influence of excellence was simply worldwide.[11]

Unfortunately, Red never got to revisit with his former surgical student.
Dr. Rabani was killed by the Taliban several years later.

Bertz and Duke would end up working together in Houston at the
medical school in its early days. "I'll never forget working nights in the
hospital and grabbing a quick bite to eat in the cafeteria. I'd watch him
take a baked potato, scoop out much of the potato while adding jalapeños with lots of the pepper juice. He'd eat what was primarily the potato's skin doused with fiery peppers."

One day, remembers Bertz, potato skins and jalapeños were not on
the menu.

It was the early 1980s, and he came rushing in my office and
told me to put my coat on and go to lunch with him. I told him
I was just too busy and he said, "Damn it, Bud (everyone got
a nickname), get your coat on." Next thing I know I'm sitting
at lunch with George H. Bush and Barbara, Ronald Reagan
and Nancy, and Bob and Elizabeth Dole. Red had treated one
of President Reagan's Secret Service detail and got the invite.
I stood there after lunch for twenty minutes watching him
converse and carry on like a member of the family. Red Duke
could be at home with presidents and paupers alike. It made
no difference. He loved people.[12]

Red's propensity for mischief surfaced on a trip to Pittsburgh with
Bertz to look at a new air ambulance program. "We pulled into a parking lot at the hospital and Red asked the parking attendant for direc-
tions. Red's query was delivered in his trademark Texas drawl, and the
parking attendant was clearly perplexed, asking, 'Where in hell are you
from?' Red without hesitation replied in his thickest Southern accent,

'Vermont.'"[13]

The Vermont prank worked much better on the hospital parking attendant than it did a few years earlier when Red tried it at a ritzy West Coast dinner in the home of William Longmire Jr., a prominent surgeon and chairman of surgery at UCLA. Longmire and his wife were hosting Nobel laureate Linus Pauling along with Indy 500 legend Andy Granatelli. Red was given specific instructions for dress code and arrival time. Tonight he was about to find himself hopelessly entangled in his own prank.

I hadn't been in Houston long when I got a call from Hollywood, California, with a request to give a lecture on nutrition and cancer, which I knew a little bit about but not much. Aside from the talk, Longmire asked, "Would you like to come to my house for dinner on Saturday night for Linus Pauling?" And I was like, "Yeah, I'd like to." An old country boy like me going to get to meet a Nobel laureate. And damned if I didn't get on an airplane and sit down with Dr. Longmire, who was one of the granddaddies, great-granddaddies of surgery in those days. We had a nice visit out there. We got there on time, landed with no trouble, and I went to the hotel and started to clean up, and turned on the television. And there was Willie Nelson on Austin City Limits going through the "Red Headed Stranger," you know, that whole damned thing.

I sat down and watched it. I kind of got lost in space, you know, and then I realized I'd gotten myself in trouble with the clock. Well, anyway, I got dressed and went to the house dressed as I'd been instructed. And they opened the door and—you know, you'd think for a dinner for Linus Pauling you'd have a bunch. Well, there was not a bunch! There were only eleven people invited. I was late and the odd man out. I never will forget the sick feeling I had. I looked across the room and there was one empty chair, and it turned out it was next to the hostess. So I go in and sit down. I try to be as inconspicuous as possible. And she was kind of a nervous ninny, you know, wanted to, I guess, cover up her nervousness for me being late and said, "Well, Dr. Duke, where are you from?" I said, "Vermont," foolish that I am. She then asked, "What town?" Well, my best buddy in the Army was from Barre, Vermont, which apparently has a lot of tungsten—they got it in that granite mountain. It was the only town I knew in Vermont so I said, "Barre." And she says, "Where? Barre, Vermont? Oh, I have many friends in Barre. Do you know . . .?" Well, when you find yourself in a hole, it's best to quit digging—but I didn't. I realized I'd gotten pretty deep and to this day I don't know how I got out of that mess. But it just goes to show she didn't bite the hook; she swallowed it and I was backpedaling all the way out the door.[14]

While Red could backpedal when he needed to, for the most part he was in fast-forward on the job and tireless in surgery and in teaching a few "young 'uns" along the way. Skilled perseverance and dedication to his patients are attributes his students and faculty colleagues commonly cite in describing him. Just a year before his death, as he ate his breakfast in the kitchen of his daughter's farmhouse, he put down his fork and got serious about the medical students of today:

The current student is a product of our culture, and they are not as a whole motivated toward unselfish commitment to the well-being of the patient. If you take, for instance, the trauma residency, they have even written papers on this. One of the things that is kind of sad is they talk about damage control. Have you ever heard of that term? When you get into a big mess like taking out part of their liver [and you] start to get in trouble because the patient is getting hypertensive, [in the past] you stopped, got control, let the patient catch up, and then kept going [to complete the procedure at hand]. Nowadays they will pack them with a jillion laparotomy pads and try to bring them back later [for a second surgery]. That is called damage control. There is a place for that, but it is not damn near every time. It has gotten to the point where some surgeons only do half an operation. Many do not take ownership. Whoever the first one is that operates on you, it would be a rare bird that he would be the second one to do it or the third, maybe the fourth. But they pass them around, and that is not good care. There is no way I can operate on somebody and then tell you about it and you have a real complete understanding like I do of the circumstances. You can see how that can get diluted when you keep doing this.[15]

Working with Red Duke always involved a few hidden sermons on patient follow-through and perseverance. More than a few of his surgical students remember his Duke-speak directive: "You take them, you raise them."

For the students who responded to his stock question, "Who's the most important person in this OR?" by answering "the surgeon" rather than "the patient," a reprimand that would make Red's irascible father proud was soon to follow. Linda Mobley, a veteran nurse who worked beside Red for years, recalls, "I'd see the new residents tell Dr. Duke that the surgeon was the most important person in the room and just cringe behind my mask as he spared no mercy reprimanding [them]. Working with Red was always, without compromise, giving your best and putting your patient first."[16]

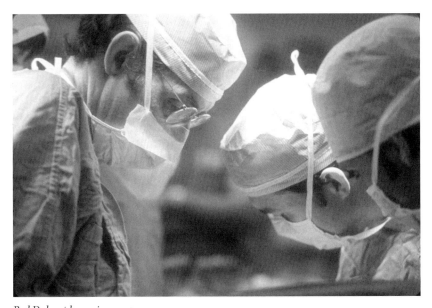

Red Duke at home in surgery.

In surgery Red could entertain, teach, and pontificate on the problems of the world without missing a beat on the procedure at hand. Country music might be playing and the atmosphere relaxed, but he was dead serious when it came to attention to detail.

His Seldin training in internal medicine married to practiced skills with the scalpel gave him a reputation for saving patients others considered beyond hope. He could bark at a team member and call someone out in strong language when occasion arose, but generally he approached the teachable moment with a constructive message.

Many veteran surgeons marveled at his ability to work long hours, far longer than most. One surgery stands out as his longest—fifty-four hours. "Yes, fifty-four hours without sleep." The procedure was not typical, fortunately. The victim was a deputy constable serving papers on a member of the criminal element in Houston when things went wrong.

> And somebody shot him right here with a shotgun [pointing to his belly button]. His belly was full of green stuff. I honestly believe that guy had eaten a quart of guacamole. And it hit the vena cava and his duodenum and pancreas—bad injury. So, hell, what do you do? And then when you have a pancreas and duodenum that messed up, and you take that out—you take out the duodenum, the head of the pancreas, and then you're supposed to put it all back together so that the bile drains into the jejunum. . . . And because he was so contaminated, I decided to remove his entire pancreas which is not that hard to do, [but] if that connection between the pancreas and the jejunum leaks, you got a mess.[17]

In telling the story Red was lost in the moment, describing intricate details of the epic procedure while simultaneously sketching on a napkin his approach and multiple complications along the way. Clearly he was not going to give up on his patient and did not (the patient survived, as best he remembered). Why attempt such a long procedure? "Yes, that's crazy, but there wasn't anybody else to do it."

For many procedures, improvisation and bucking the status quo were not out of the question. Afghanistan, the army, and the Boy Scouts had taught him that if you don't have what you need, you make

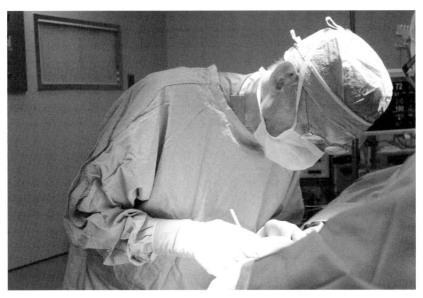

Red Duke at work in the trauma suites of Memorial Hermann Hospital–Texas Medical Center.

do. For years Red's surgical residents would hear him preaching during surgery on the value of leeches and maggots for cleaning wounds and brown sugar to promote healing. One surprised resident was sent from the operating room to the grocery store during a long surgical procedure to buy additional brown sugar. "Brown sugar, not white sugar," Red yelled out the door as his student headed for the store scratching his head.[18] It worked time after time, and Red rejoiced in proving his point. He also pointed to support in the medical literature for the position that alternative medicine should not necessarily be dismissed out of hand.

Looking back, Red summed up his teaching career with satisfaction. "I've had some really great students over the years, and I can proudly say not a one was taught to do half a surgery or to think of anything beyond the patient as the focus of everything we do."[19]

CHAPTER 19
Saying Good-bye

Step back in time to early April 2013. Red Duke was alive and well and hurrying about the hospital and medical school, meeting and greeting everybody who crossed his path. On the news one morning he had learned that Margaret Thatcher, Britain's Iron Lady, had died of a stroke at eighty-seven. Her death had given him pause. Red himself was eighty-four and feeling fine—at least for the moment.

The evening ahead was one he had been looking forward to for some time. His former chairman and surgical colleague, Stanley Dudrick, was in town for an annual lecture scheduled the next morning. The dinner that night at a local restaurant would be a chance to hash over old times with him and a number of the surgery department's alumni. They could revisit the early days when Dudrick first arrived in Houston and when he sought Red out in Afghanistan. Dudrick was one of the few people who called Red by his first name, James or Jim.

Dudrick in recent years had retired as chairman emeritus of surgery at the Yale-affiliated St. Mary's Hospital in Waterbury, Connecticut, where the surgical department had been named for him. Now he was coming home to the Texas Medical Center. The event was special, and Dudrick remembers the evening in precise detail. It did not turn out well.

> My birthday is April ninth, and the Dudrick Lecture was given every April ninth as a birthday present. . . . The residents and the alumni that we had trained were the prime movers for the event. I know it must have been April eighth that Jim and I were at the dinner. We had a lovely dinner because we were all telling stories and probably embellishing them all with each other. There were pictures to share, laughter, jokes, and endless stories of memorable experiences. As the evening wore on we knew we had to be back at seven o'clock in the morning

for a lecture, and each of us around the table got up and said something. That's what I liked the best—everybody got up and said something.

Then, as people were leaving, we were saying bye to them. . . . We both walked down the stairs of the restaurant and then out the front, and at every opportunity we'd stop for a minute to talk some more. It took a long time to get from the top of the stairs to his pickup. But it must have been around ten thirty we said good night. We were the only two left there. Terry [Dudrick's wife] was waiting by the car, and all the rest of them were gone. Jim got in his pickup and left.

I got called perhaps at four in the morning to let me know that Jim was in the operating room and not as the surgeon. I was told that he had an infarction in the heart, and it was at the point in the heart where the attachments of the heart valves to the little muscular strips that hold the valve in place attach to the wall of the heart. When that infarcted, that one or two strands and muscles tore away from the wall . . . and that's very often fatal, because it mechanically just, as you can imagine, screws up flow and heart. It rips up the red cells, a lot of stuff.

At any rate, we got a report that Jim was still in a recovery room, doing okay, but it was tenuous. We had a moment of prayer for him, hoping that everything was going to come out okay. We did hear by the time we left Houston the next day that he was out of the woods but had a long row to hoe. And then I called down there every day to talk to people to find out how he was coming along, and he was making progress

Typical Red, I heard that a week after surgery he insisted on giving a lecture he was scheduled to give, and they put him in a wheelchair and wheeled him to the lecture hall. He apparently gave a lecture from the wheelchair to the students about one week post op. That's the James Duke I knew and recruited so many years ago.[1]

Actually, Red had driven back to the hospital and parked his truck in a nearby parking garage when he first felt a problem. Back in his call room he lay down and later told Sara, "It felt like an elephant was sitting on my chest. Figured ol' Red better get checked out." As he walked into the ER, a new admissions clerk did not recognize him and asked if he came by ambulance or car. "No, I just walked," he replied, trying to defeat the medical issue at hand with humor.

Red was in dire straits and remembered few details beyond his admission. It was not until after surgery that he asked for his family to be notified. Sara received a call early the next morning. "Typical of my dad, he told them to wait until after the surgery so not to wake me up." She left College Station immediately, notifying family members along the way.

Thanks to the surgical skills of his colleagues, Red survived against the odds. But the heart attack had done its damage; his strength and energy were drained, never to return. And Red would never return to the operating room as the surgeon. Vulnerable as he was now, he found that what he really wanted was to be with family. It was the family he had set aside for the most part in recent years, but although their tie had been strained, it had never been cut. With one of their number wounded, the others materialized and closed ranks around him.

Looking into Sara's face, especially her eyes, you see her father. You see his intellect and his straightforward approach to the world. It was to the peace and sanity of her hundred-year-old farmhouse, with its chicken coops and gardens and its chorus of barking dogs, that Red went to finish out as much as he could of the last year of his life. His children helped him, and so did Betty. At last he was able to focus on them in ways they had always wanted him to but that had not been possible during the decades when he had been married to the hospital, the cameras, the distant mountains, the big guns.

The transition to College Station had been easy. In the hospital Red had said he "lived like a coyote." Moving him from his hospital digs to Sara's house required only a wheelchair and a handful of hospital scrubs (which he continued to wear), the growing array of his medications, and the calendar of medical appointments that Sara and Charles monitored.

Here I came on weekends for my breakfasts with Red. I wrote a piece called "Country Breakfast with Red Duke" to bring the medical community in Houston up to date on him. It became one of the most requested reprints in my four decades of writing.[2] These breakfast stories, collected week after week during the six months he was in College Station, took on growing importance to both of us, although Red knew he would never read the book that would be based on them. Some breakfast meetings ended with an invitation to come back the next day, if old friends were dropping by to talk. Needless to say, I was there.

His stories reliving his seminary days and his discovery of Albert Schweitzer revealed that he had never seen film footage of Schweitzer working in his African clinic. I laid hands on a video disk that contained old film shot in the clinic in the 1950s and brought it on my laptop one morning to show Red.[3] There in the kitchen, as Sara broke fresh eggs into a hot skillet, Red's eyes intently followed Schweitzer into the primitive clinic, with its tin roof and plywood floors, to examine a patient. Behind Schweitzer was an old wooden shelf with a handful of brown bottles containing all the drugs the great doctor had to offer.

"Damn," Red said, "he didn't have much to work with." He was glued to Schweitzer's beautiful white head and compassionate face. For Red it was visual confirmation of something he had always known—that often words of comfort and the touch of a hand are more powerful than the most potent medicine on the shelf.

· · ·

Not long after Red had gone to live with Sara, when he still appeared to be improving, a new elementary school was named after him in Manvel, south of Houston. He was invited to attend the dedication. This was one of the few public appearances Red made after his heart attack, but (against the advice of some) he was determined to go. Moreover, he intended to fly in on Life Flight and land in the parking lot to give the students a thrill. The helicopter lifted off from Hermann with him and Sara aboard, but the pilot saw a storm brewing ahead and was forced back to the hospital. Red was unloaded in his wheelchair, but, undismayed, he and Sara got into a car and started off again. This put them an hour and a half late for the dedication, but no one seemed to mind. When he arrived, the whole school stood and applauded as he was wheeled into the auditorium.

Sitting in his wheelchair, frail but quick-witted, Red was once again the star of the show. The audience could hardly contain its delight as

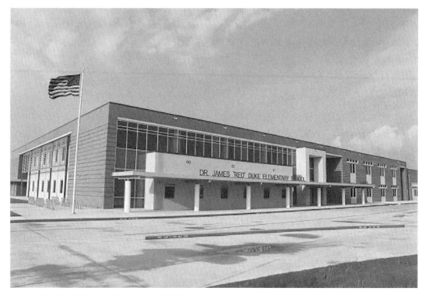

James H. "Red" Duke Elementary School.

he recounted his own years in elementary school. "To this day," he told them, "I can remember when Miss Tinsley would call me in that voice of reprimand, 'Little Boy!' or the dreaded full-name treatment, 'James Henry Duke!' It still sends a shiver up my spine to think about it."[4]

In the audience that morning, students, teachers, and parents alike laughed in sympathy—and empathy—with their hero and school namesake.

Back home at Sara's, life was quieter. Jake was a reliable source of affection and entertainment. He was a regular interloper at breakfast. He would stop by the table for a bite of sausage that Red would cut from his plate with a surgeon's precision and send flying wide and high over the coffee cups to be inhaled in midflight by man's best friend. Red kept a box of Jake's treats handy among his growing array of medications on a TV tray in the family room. Here we sometimes just sat quietly and watched television together as Jake nosed around for a treat or sat with his head on Red's knee or under his hand. Red's hearing was as bad as ever, so the TV was loud as he searched out anything on it that related to Alaska, the great outdoors, and wildlife. The taller and the more majestic the mountains, the deeper the snow, the better.

But more often we talked. I noticed that when Red told a story he sometimes lingered over Betty's part in it. He especially liked to talk about the Alaskan trip they had made together in their youth. As I watched Betty weaving her path through his memories, I realized how indelibly their thirty years together had stamped her into his life. It was clear to me that in their old age Red Duke still loved the mother of his children. The two now talked frequently by phone.

"When Red became so sick and was in College Station," Betty told me later, "we came back together. We talked often and we always ended every call with 'I love you,' and 'I love you, too.'"[5] Betty had moved to a house in Cedar Park (near Austin), but with Red living at Sara's, she started staying at the old house at New Ulm farm. It was a shorter drive to College Station, and she could make day-trips there to be with him.

His convalescence at Sara's ended when he had to go back to the Texas Medical Center because he needed more consistent physical therapy and more blood work for pulmonary monitoring than could be provided at home. Although his mind remained sharp, his body grew steadily weaker. Here was Red Duke's other family, his medical family— the doctors and nurses, the Life Flight team, the assorted health professionals and support staff who had worked with him for years, some of them his former students. Two nurses who stuck especially close to him now were Linda Mobley and Patty Read. Sometimes they brought Jake by for a visit.

On good days they would wheel Red out to a waiting car and take him to dinner. They liked giving him a break from hospital life, and since living at the hospital was no longer optional, he liked getting a break from it, too. "When we couldn't go out, he'd sometimes ask for his favorite soup or dish from this restaurant or that. The whole community cared, and the son of the owner of one restaurant he frequented near the medical center would run Red's favorite soup over on short order whenever we called."[6]

In time the opportunities to leave the hospital or to spend a moment with Jake came to an end. Red was moved to the intensive care unit, and there the atmosphere was very different from Sara's house. Machines beeped and instruments ticked off the numbers of life as intensive-care nurses monitored them at the bedside. There was a gravity in the air that made good spirits hard even to pretend to find.

But Red still had a reward or two left for a visitor. I had recently gone to Hillsboro and made a slide show of images from his childhood that he watched with absorption on my laptop. The finale of the show was a shot that brought a grin to his face. His famous mustache was now thin and gray, but it still had a dance or two left in it for the Hill County courthouse. "Ain't she beautiful," he beamed. Another slide showed close-ups of the granite markers outside the courthouse. He had me read them all, word for word. I misread a date, and astonishingly, he corrected me.

Spotting the alley next to Bond's drugstore, he squinted as if trying to see far into the shadows, where he had folded newspapers on many a predawn morning before he and his high school buddies set off on their separate trecks through the town. Hillsboro was a world he had been glad enough to leave behind in a literal sense, but in spirit he had carried it with him.

I stowed my laptop and said good-bye. At the door I turned to look back at his tired face, surrounded by tubes and monitors. He looked me in the eyes and said, "I'm tired of all this bullshit." I replied sadly, "I know."

• • •

Within two days of that visit, Red asked to be moved from the ICU back to his familiar hospital room. He no longer needed or wanted all the high-tech monitoring devices and around-the-clock interventions designed to sustain his exhausted body. With his family by his side, he was now receiving palliative care and moving through the final stages of his life. He and his family had accepted death, and it was near.

Here in his hospital suite, the monitors were replaced with the vigilant eyes and tender touch of family. Here his favorite Willie Nelson songs sometimes hung in the air. He had other country favorites, too. He told the nurses about Bobby Bare, and Linda Mobley showed up with an album and a turntable to play Bobby Bare songs for him. He knew every word. His Bible was at hand, and so were his families, both biological and medical.

This is where I came to say good-bye one last time, on the last Sunday of his life. I came to show my respect, but I stood in the back corner of the room, because this was family time. Betty was on her way from her home near Austin to be with him. I slipped back into the doorway of the adjoining suite as she came into the room and stood by his bed, gently grasping both his hands. They looked into each other's faces with full knowledge. They understood everything.

Outside was a beautiful, sunny Sunday afternoon. Inside, Betty and the children now joined forces with Red's medical family. He might have been brought into the world with the wrong name, but he was going to leave it knowing exactly who he was and how much he meant to other people.

It was an extraordinary time. Red had three days left, and he spent them in a world of love and tenderness. His body wanted to die, and he was not afraid of death, or even of dying, but still he couldn't quite do it. Patty Read, who was the nurse by his side during his last night, remembers that he said, "I know I'm going to meet Jesus; I just don't know how to let go."

The next morning, a powerful thunderstorm approached the city.

Betty remembers that morning in detail. She went to Red's side, sensing that stubborn streak she knew so well. "I leaned over and whispered in his ear, 'It's okay, Red, you can let go.'"[7] Red nodded. The man who had saved so many lives and worked on the fine edge between life and death for so many years was now on that edge himself. Red and Betty had travelled long miles together, from narrow icy routes across Alaska to death-defying roads through the treacherous passes of Afghanistan. They had left each other and they had come back. And now they were here.

Linda Mobley was in the hospital's operating theater on the second floor.

> I heard thunder in the operating room. I worked with Red for seventeen years and I have never heard thunder in the OR before or since that day. I just knew. I turned to my colleagues and said, "It's time. I have to go." I rushed to his room. We took his blood pressure and he opened his eyes and winked at me and said, "It's time." That's when we called in the family and palliative care team. He said, "There's a wave. I can feel it from head to toe." I said, "Ride that wave, Red."[8]

Patricia remembers her brother's eyes turning to the left as the rain outside pounded the window. "He saw something," she says, "and said very clearly, with no uncertainty, 'Praise the Lord.'"[9]

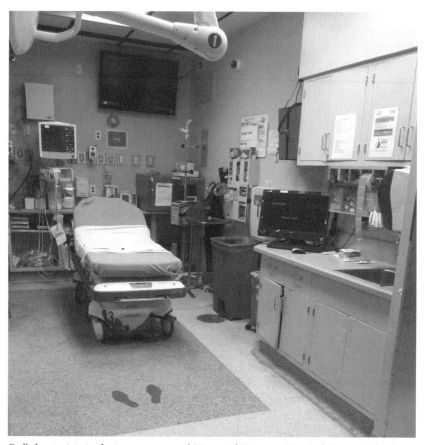

Red's boot prints in the trauma rooms of Memorial Hermann Hospital–Texas Medical Center (in red, of course). Courtesy of Dwight C. Andrews.

Casey Slusher, one of the palliative care team, adds, "I remember he wanted to hear hymns and asked to hear the Lord's Prayer."[10] Those in the room gathered close as the words of Matthew 6:9–13 brought their familiar comfort. Hallie remembers that at the end of the prayer her father provided his own closure, when he was ready, with a final "Amen."[11]

He closed his eyes. They gathered tightly around him, both families together as one. It was 4:12 p.m. on the afternoon of Wednesday, August 25, 2015.

Outside, the thunder stopped.

Red Duke had left the room.

Epilogue

Today the whirl of Life Flight rotors echoes across the Texas Medical Center as another patient is rushed to the trauma unit that Red Duke helped build and then nourished down through the years. Patients facing their own battles with death are rushed from the helicopter down the corridors to the waiting trauma team, many of whom trained with Red in years past and follow his protocols and example instinctively. The only difference now is that Red Duke is not standing there with a wisecrack and a scalpel to remind the medical team that "we're here to entertain the patient till God makes up his mind."

The hospital's trauma unit is now the Memorial Hermann Red Duke Trauma Institute. Red's boot prints have been painted on the floor just inside the doorway of each trauma room for all to see—in red, of course. People like to think that he is standing there in spirit, watching over every patient, every student, every caregiver.

A year after Red's death, first graders from the James H. "Red" Duke Elementary School went to the McGovern Medical School to share drawings they had made of Red Duke, their school's hero and namesake. It was his birthday, and he would have been eighty-eight that day. In a crowded hall outside the dean's office, hundreds gathered as the students displayed their art and sang happy birthday to Dr. Red Duke. Their artwork depicted a bespectacled, mustachioed doctor who stood tall while helicopters buzzed around him. It was November 16, 2016, and the medical school was again humid with tears as people who had known Red Duke were reminded of what they had lost.

Somewhere during the spring in the high country of far West Texas a tiny ewe, a newborn bighorn sheep, takes a shaky step forward while her mother watches guardedly. Such a sight would bring a wide grin to Red's face, followed by "Ain't they something." The bighorn sheep continue to grow in numbers and are symbolic of the many conservation causes that Red, Teddy Roosevelt, and other dedicated people, past and present, have invested in for future generations.

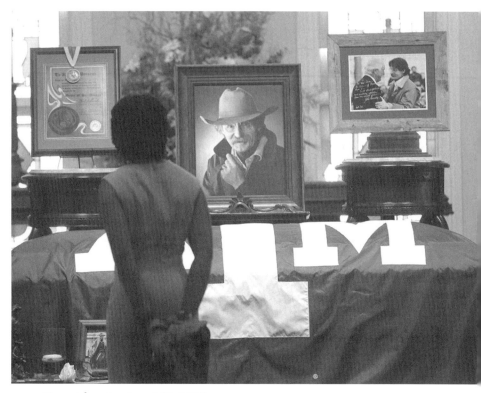

Memorial service, August 29, 2015.

Notes

Introduction

1. Today, the University of Texas System has six health components across the state. They and the dates they opened are as follows: UT Medical Branch at Galveston (1891); UT M. D. Anderson Cancer Center (Houston, 1941); UT Southwestern Medical Center (Dallas, 1949); UT Health Science Center at Houston (1972); UT Health Science Center at San Antonio (1972); and UT Health Science Center at Tyler (1977). Additional health components are being added in Austin and South Texas.

2. Those breakfasts first found their way into print when UTHealth honored Red Duke for a lifetime of service in November 2014. I wrote a piece for the occasion titled "Country Breakfast with Red Duke" that has become one of the most requested reprints in my four decades of writing. It was first posted October 31, 2014, as part of a blog series called *'Bout Time* and available online: https://www.uth.edu/blog/bout-time/.

3. *Buck James*, TriStar Television, ABC, aired September 27, 1987–May 5, 1988.

4. Texas State Cemetery, Austin, Travis County, Texas, Section: Monument Hill, Section 2 (H2); Row: R, Number: 24B.

Chapter 1

1. Red Duke, interview by William H. Kellar, September 11, 2014.

2. Ibid.

3. Mary Elizabeth "Magele" Potter to Helen Duke, December 11, 1928. Letters are hereafter cited in the text. Unless otherwise noted, they are in the family's possession.

4. Ellis County History Overview, "Ellis County's Emergence as a Leading Cotton-Producing Center," accessed January 25, 2017, http://www.rootsweb.ancestry.com/~txecm/ellis.htm. This undated research was conducted by Hardy Heck Moore Cultural Resource Consultants for the US Department of Energy.

5. Ibid., 7.

6. N. Don Macon, *Monroe Dunaway Anderson, His Legacy: A History of the Texas Medical Center, 50th Anniversary Edition* (Houston: Texas Medical Center, 1994).

7. *Ennis Daily News*, November 17, 1932.

8. Ibid., June 17, 1932. Red appeared onstage with Teddy Norman, Peggy Cox, Jimmie Estelle Sims, and Earl Shaw Jr.

9. Event program, "The Little Cabaret in Smiles of 1933," a production of McCleary Sisters School of the Dance, Texas Theatre, Dallas, Texas, June 17, 1932.

10. Red Duke, interview by the author, September 17, 2014. Interviews with Red Duke and members of his family are by the author unless otherwise noted. All such interviews (transcripts and/or recordings) are in the author's possession.

11. *Ennis Daily News*, 1936, undated clippings.

12. Red Duke, interview by the author, September 17, 2014.

13. American Association for Pediatric Ophthalmology and Strabismus, "Strabismus," https:/www.aapos.org/terms/conditions/100.

14. Red Duke, interview by the author, September 11, 2014.

15. Ibid., personal conversation with the author, September 10, 2014.

16. Ibid., interview by the author, October 10, 2014.

17. Ibid., February 20, 2015.

18. "J. Henry Duke Given Buffet Supper by Tab. Young People," *Ennis Daily News*, May 29, 1937.

Chapter 2

1. T. Lindsay Baker, *Gangster Tour of Texas* (College Station: Texas A&M University Press, 2011), 43.

2. *Images of America: Hillsboro*, edited by the Hillsboro Heritage Society (Charleston: Arcadia, 2013), 2.

3. Ibid., 10.

4. Ibid., 14.

5. Tommy West, "When Patrons Were 'Guests,'" *Texas Business*, December 1976.

6. Robert A. Rieder, "Electric Interurban Railways," *Handbook of Texas Online*, accessed January 25, 2017, http://www.tshaonline.org/handbook/online/articles/eqe12.

7. Patti Carlton, email message to the author, May 26, 2016.

8. Red Duke, interview by the author, February 20, 2015.

9. Ibid., high school essay, untitled, undated.

10. The author used Ancestry.com to construct Red Duke's family tree. Records used included birth certificates, census data, voter registration records, and other documents. Additionally, family members provided personal documents and photos. All family history in this book is derived from these resources.

11. Red Duke, interview by the author, February 20, 2015. Red noted that Grandpa Cherry "got busy and bought some mules and dragline scoop. He started building roads and bought some land because that land didn't cost anything out

around Brownwood. Apparently, he said the group of men that he'd been working with up there got into some hard times, and one of 'em got killed, so they broke up, and it was apparently the James Gang."

12. Patricia Hipps, interview by the author, February 25, 2016.

13. Red Duke, interview by the author, September 17, 2015. Red noted, "But this John Simmons apparently abused Dad a whole lot, and he went to live with his grandpa Cherry." Accounts of Henry's abuse come from multiple family members, among whom there is a consensus that Henry turned his resulting rage and "brutal" behavior on his own family, with lasting, negative effects on his children and his grandchildren. Helen Duke protected Henry's image as the responsible, community-minded Baptist deacon that he appeared in public to be. But inside his home, he was a very different man, whose anger and constant tirades and bad behavior haunt his extended family in many ways to this day.

14. Betty Duke Kent, interview by the author, February 25, 2016.

Chapter 3

1. Patricia Hipps, interview by the author, February 25, 2016.

2. Ibid.

3. Red Duke, personal conversation with the author, February 20, 2015.

4. Ibid., interview by William H. Kellar, September 11, 2014.

5. Patricia Hipps, interview by the author, February 25, 2016.

6. Red Duke, interview by the author, October 10, 2014. Red added, "They could pick four rows at a time. Generally I would try to pick two just crawling along."

7. *Hillsboro Daily Mirror*, clipping, hand dated 1942.

8. Boy Scouts of America website, "The Scout Law," http://www.scouting.org/ scoutsource/venturing/about/welcome.aspx.

9. See the National Eagle Scout Association's website: http://www.nesa.org/ distinguishedaward.html. Red Duke earned his Eagle Scout rank August 16, 1946, and was awarded distinguished status on January 16, 1975.

10. Red Duke, interview by William H. Kellar, May 22, 2012.

11. Ibid., interview by the author, October 10, 2014.

12. Robert Peterson, "The Man Who Got Lost in the Fog," *Scouting* (October 2001), http://scoutingmagazine.org/issues/0110/d-wwas.html.

13. *Boys' Life*, July 15, 1916, 22.

14. Ibid.

15. Boy Scouts of America website, "Theodore Roosevelt," http://www .scouting.org/RTN/History/TRoosevelt.aspx.

16. Red Duke, interview by the author, September 17, 2014. Red recalled one of his father's half brothers, a Simmons, who did go to college. "That son came to live

with us when we were living in Ennis, and he'd never seen a football, but he was good at it, and he apparently got a scholarship. I've still got sweaters—Texas Tech football sweaters. He was the first guy in that part of the family that I know who went to college, and he's the only one who graduated before I did. He lived in the building where they generated the heat. . . . When he graduated, he continued to stay there for a little while. Something went wrong with the pumps. He went down into the reservoir to fix it. The feeling was he was overcome by the fumes and drowned."

Chapter 4

1. *Hillsboro Evening Mirror*, "111 Receive College, High School Diplomas Monday," May 28, 1946, 1.

2. Betty Duke Kent, telephone conversation with the author, November 2017.

3. Red Duke, telephone conversation with the author, February 26, 2015.

4. Ibid., interview by William H. Kellar, May 22, 2012.

5. Ibid.

6. Ibid., interview by the author, March 6, 2015.

7. Texas A&M University, "History of the University," retrieved January 30, 2017, http://www.tamu.edu/about/history.html.

8. Ibid.

9. Gil Gilchrist, "A Message from the President," November 7, 1946.

10. Rose Cahalan, "Celebrating 100 Years of Bevo and Getting to Know the Newest Steer to Hold the Title," *Texas Alcalde*, September 2016, 39.

11. Agricultural and Mechanical College of Texas, grade report for first semester (fall) 1946/1947 for James Henry Duke Jr. Mailed by H. L. Heaton, registrar, to Mr. J. H. Duke, 909 E. Franklin, Hillsboro, Texas.

12. The university's president, Gibb Gilchrist, also noted in his November 7, 1946, Message from the President the unusual circumstances of the time for incoming freshmen like Red. "Like all colleges in the nation, A. and M. College had an unprecedented enrollment in September. Of the total enrollment two-thirds, or more than 6,000 are veterans of World War II. Prior to September, realizing that facilities would be overtaxed, enrollment was limited so that all Texas veterans who were entering College for the first time, all former students of the College, and all June graduates of Texas high schools would have a place at A. and M. The quota of Freshmen was quickly reached; so in order to care for additional students, the Bryan Army Air Field was secured and converted into the A. and M. College Annex for overflow Freshmen."

13. Marion P. Bowden was a Lt. Col., Inf., Tactical Officer filing the report from the Office of the Commandant to the Assistant Dean of Men, Agricultural and Mechanical College of Texas, May 25, 1949. Subject: Dog in Dorm 2.

14. Ibid., report, May 25, 1949. Subject: Student Behavior: James H. Duke, N. R. Patterson.

15. Red Duke to family, February 16, 1949. This letter illustrates an upbeat Red Duke during his senior year, when military life and improving grades demonstrate his growth and his success as a senior preparing for graduation. "I've been what some people call busy, but I'd say that [is] an understatement. I've got a contract [armored division] and thus far I'm just eating it up. I really get a buzz out of those tanks." As for grades, he notes exams were going well with all A's and B's—"all pulled up from mid-semester by one letter."

16. "The Yell Leaders: How Texas A&M's Loudest Tradition Got Its Start," Texas A&M University, http://www.myaggienation.com/history_traditions/yell_leaders/.

17. Red Duke, interview by the author, September 11, 2014.

18. The story was told at Red Duke's family memorial service during eulogies. Service held at the Jasek Chapel, Geo. H. Lewis & Sons, Houston, August 29, 2015.

19. Hallie Duke, telephone conversation with the author, January 17, 2017.

20. C. C. Munroe, "Duke Is One of Seven Outstanding at Hood," *The Battalion*, August 1, 1949.

21. Frederick L. Briuer, "Fort Hood," *The Handbook of Texas*, last modified January 3, 2017, https://tshaonline.org/handbook/online/articles/qbf25.

22. C. C. Munroe, "Duke Is One of Seven Outstanding at Hood."

Chapter 5

1. I found seven letters that during the summer of 1951 were exchanged among Red, his pastor in Hillsboro, and Dr. Alfred Carpenter, director of the chaplains commission, Home Mission Board, Southern Baptist Convention, Atlanta, in an effort get Red discharged from active duty to return to seminary and prepare for the chaplaincy. There was a shortage of chaplains serving the army, but the process of switching into the chaplaincy was nevertheless complicated. Red's first request is dated June 1, 1951, to Dr. Carpenter. In a letter dated August 17, 1951, Dr. Carpenter certified Red's status as "a bona fide Southern Baptist minister." Red could only wait to see if he would be released from active duty to return to seminary. He wrote home on August 24 that the certificate from Carpenter made a lump in his throat and added, "I have taken the necessary steps to forward this letter through channels although I am getting a good dose of what red tape is. . . . All we can do now is hope and pray." The release he sought was never forthcoming.

2. "History of Fort Knox," http://www.knox.army.mil/about/history.aspx.

3. Red Duke, interview by William H. Kellar, May 22, 2012.

4. "Camp Kilmer," National Archives, New York City. https://www.archives.gov/nyc/exhibit/camp-kilmer.

5. A letter from Henry to Red in Germany dated February 3, 1952, is part of the endless search for the right set of china for Red to purchase for his mother. In the letter, Henry notes he had driven to Dallas to look at china patterns at Neiman

Marcus but none matched the pictures Red had sent, although some sets in Dallas were closing out at half the original price. Henry suggested that Red buy three saucers of the ones he liked and send them to Hillsboro so Henry and Helen could make a better decision. Henry's plan was "we still won't tell Mother that you are actually buying her a set." A letter one week later changed the plan again.

Chapter 6

1. Red Duke, interview by the author, March 6, 2015.

2. Ibid.

3. Betty Duke Kent, personal conversation with the author, February 25, 2016.

4. Red Duke, interview by the author, February 12, 2014.

5. Betty Duke Kent, interview by the author, January 8, 2016.

6. Ibid., personal conversation with the author, February 3, 2016.

7. Ibid.

8. Jeremy Pelzer, "Gordon Cowden's Last Words of Love Remembered during First Service for Colorado Theatre Shooting Victims," *New York Daily News*, July 25, 2012.

9. Betty Duke Kent, interview by the author, March 1, 2017.

10. Ibid.

11. Ibid., December 22, 2016.

12. Ibid.

13. Red Duke, interview by the author, December 12, 2014.

14. George Seaver, *Albert Schweitzer: The Man and His Mind*, 4th ed. (London: Adam & Charles Black, 1955), 222–24; and James Brabazon, *Albert Schweitzer: A Biography* (New York: Syracuse University Press, 2000), 92.

Chapter 7

1. Red Duke, personal conversation with the author, March 6, 2015.

2. Betty Duke Kent, interview by the author, January 8, 2016.

3. George H. Cockburn, "Frontier College in Action," undated handout used by the college to orient new "labourer-teachers" like Red before arrival in Canada. The single page handout includes a personal note: "George H. Cockburn was associated with Frontier College as a labourer-teacher in the early thirties. He is a graduate of the University of British Columbia and of Toronto—a man of sound ideals and purposeful in life."

4. Alfred Fitzpatrick, *The University in Overalls*, paperback edition (n.p.: Bibliobazaar, 2009), 121.

5. Red Duke, daily log prepared for Frontier College, June 22, 1953–July 19, 1953. This typed summary of his work in Canada includes twenty-seven workdays. Red Duke family papers.

6. E. W. Robinson to James H. Duke, October 24, 1956, family personal papers. This letter from the principal of the college to Red in Fort Worth notes, "We have not had much reason or opportunity for correspondence with you of late but we often think of the fine contribution you made to Frontier College and Canada's camp-men. . . . We are recruiting winter staff Labourer-teachers. This is no easy task."

Chapter 8

1. Betty Duke Kent, telephone conversation with the author, March 1, 2017.

2. "Tornado Slashes Wide Path of Death and Destruction," *Dallas Times Herald*, April 3, 1957.

3. Red Duke, interview by William Kellar, May 22, 2012.

4. Course Catalog 1956/1957, UT Southwestern Medical School, Dallas, Texas. Health Sciences Digital Library and Learning Center, UT Southwestern Medical Center. A full set of course catalogs (1943–present) can be found in the Health Sciences Digital Library and Learning Center, UT Southwestern Medical Center.

5. UT Southwestern Medical Center, Mission and History, "History," http://www.utsouthwestern.edu/about-us/mission-history/.

6. 75 Years of Vision: Part 1: 1939–1979, *Southwestern Medical Perspectives*, spring 2014, 16.

7. Ibid, 36.

8. Ibid, 39.

9. Ibid, 41.

10. Course Catalog 1956/1957, UT Southwestern Medical School, Dallas, Texas, 23.

11. Freshman Schedule: 1957/1958. UT Southwestern Medical School Health Sciences Digital Library and Learning Center, UT Southwestern Medical Center. Red's freshman schedule was published for the terms Fall (September 9–December 1, 1957), Winter Part I and II (December 21–February 8, 1958), and Winter Part III (February 10–March 8, 1958). Red's simplified block schedule can also be found in the Course Catalog 1956/1957 for the three twelve-week terms, with listings provided for his freshman and sophomore years.

12. Betty Duke Kent, telephone conversation with the author, March 1, 2017.

13. Red Duke, interview by the author, September 11, 2014.

14. "Med Student Dies in Dallas Collision," *Dallas Morning News*, January 30, 1957.

15. Betty Duke Kent, telephone conversation with the author, March 1, 2017.

16. Ibid.

17. Course Catalog 1956/1957, UT Southwestern Medical School, Dallas. Health Sciences Digital Library and Learning Center, UT Southwestern Medical Center.

18. Kay Ponder, "Branches of the University: Southwestern Medical School," *The Daily Texan*, 2.

19. Red Duke, interview by the author, September 11, 2014.

20. "75 Years of Vision: Part 1: 1939–1979," *Southwestern Medical Perspectives*, spring 2014, 35. The Southwestern Medical Foundation notes that in 1951, within a few months after Seldin arrived, "the Chairman of Pediatrics left for Rochester, the Chairman of Surgery (and Dean) left for Washington University in St. Louis and the Chairman of Obstetrics and Gynecology left for the University of Illinois. By the end of 1951, not a single full-time chairman remained in any clinical department."

21. Lori Stahl, "Dr. Donald W. Seldin Recognized with Plaza Named in His Honor," *Center Times*, UT Southwestern Medical Center, accessed March 27, 2017, http://www.utsouthwestern.edu/newsroom/center-times/year-2014/june-july/donald-seldin.html.

22. William Clifford Roberts, "Donald Wayne Seldin, MD: A Conversation with the Editor," interview, *Baylor University Medical Center Proceedings* 16 (2003), 195.

23. Red Duke, interview by William H. Kellar, May 22, 2012.

24. William Clifford Roberts, "Donald Wayne Seldin, MD," 194–95.

25. Ibid, 209.

26. Course Catalog 1960/1961, "Degrees Conferred May 30, 1960." University of Texas Southwestern Medical School, Dallas. Health Sciences Digital Library and Learning Center, UT Southwestern Medical Center.

27. Match Day is held once a year in the spring for all the medical schools in the country. On that day seniors find out which medical school they have been "matched" to for their postdoctoral (residency) training. They have interviewed around the country and specified their preferences. On this day they all find out where they will be going. Match Day is an event, and families attend. Each student gets an envelope, and they all open their envelopes at the same time. This is a big tradition for seniors as they enter the next phase of their medical lives.

28. Testimony of Dr. George T. Shires, *Report of the Warren Commission on the Assassination of President Kennedy* (New York: McGraw-Hill, 1964), online at http://mcadams.posc.mu.edu/russ./testimony/shires.htm.

29. Red Duke, interview by the author, September 11, 2014.

30. Stanley Dudrick, email message to the author, December 19, 2016.

31. Ibid.

32. Tim O'Neil, "A Look Back—The Jungle Doctor, Tom Dooley, Succumbs to Cancer in 1961," *St. Louis Post-Dispatch*, January 18, 2014.

33. Red Duke, personal conversation with the author, September 18, 2014.

34. Tim O'Neil, "A Look Back."

35. Robert Shaw, quoted by Red Duke, personal conversation with the author, September 11, 2014.

Chapter 9

1. Testimony of Dr. George T. Shires, *Report of the Warren Commission on the Assassination of President Kennedy*, http://mcadams.posc.mu.edu/russ./testimony/shires.htm.

2. Red Duke, interview by the author, September 17, 2014.

3. Testimony of Dr. Robert Shaw, *Report of the Warren Commission*.

4. Ibid.

5. Red Duke, personal conversation with the author, September 17, 2014.

6. Betty Duke Kent, telephone conversation with the author, December 14, 2016.

Chapter 10

1. Red Duke, interview by the author, February 21, 2015.

2. Ibid., interview by William H. Kellar, May 22, 2012.

3. Ibid.

4. John C. Esposito, *Fire in the Grove: The Cocoanut Grove Tragedy and Its Aftermath* (Boston: Da Capo, 2006), 226.

5. Erica Goode, "Dr. Francis Moore, 88, Dies; Innovative Leader in Surgery," *New York Times*, November 29, 2001.

6. Francis D. Moore, *Metabolic Care of the Surgical Patient* (Philadelphia: W. B. Saunders, 1959).

7. Red Duke, interview by the author, September 11, 2014.

8. Ibid., interview by William H. Kellar, May 22, 2012.

9. Contract between Parkland Memorial Hospital and James H. Duke Jr., MD, as a first year resident in surgery, July 1, 1961–June 30, 1962. "The Party of the First Part agrees to pay the Party of the Second Part a monthly allowance of $75." Signed December 16, 1960. Duke family papers.

10. Betty Duke Kent, interview by the author, February 3, 2016.

11. Red Duke, interview by William H. Kellar, May 22, 2012.

12. Rebecca Duke, email message to the author, January 19, 2017.

13. Betty Duke Kent, personal conversation with the author, February 25, 2016.

14. Red Duke, interview by William H. Kellar, May 22, 2012.

15. Ibid.

16. Ibid.

17. Michael Sheehy, "Woodstock: How the Media Missed the Historic Angle of the Breaking Story," *Journalism History* 37, no. 4 (winter 2012).

Chapter 11

1. Red Duke, interview by William H. Kellar, May 22, 2012.

2. James Dunlap, "A Dallasite Fears for His Afghan Friends," *Dallas Morning News*, January 4, 1979.

3. Ibid.

4. H. C. Urschel Jr. and B. B. Urschel, "Robert R. Shaw, M.D.: Thoracic Surgical Hero, Afghanistan Medical Pioneer, Champion for the Patient, Never a Surgical Society President," *Annals of Thoracic Surgery*, 93, no. 6 (2012): 2111–16, https://www.ncbi.nim.nih.gov/pubmed/22632518.

5. James Dunlap, "A Dallasite Fears for His Afghan Friends."

6. Richard Hart, "The Story of Afghanistan and Loma Linda," News of the Week: Notes from the President, Loma Linda University Health, November 14, 2013, https://myllu.llu.edu/newsoftheweek/story/?id=13552. After 9/11, Loma Linda University continued to serve the Wazir Akbar Khan orthopedic hospital in Kabul. A hospital apartment complex was built on the hospital compound to provide additional security, but in 2007 the agreement was discontinued due to persistent unrest in the country.

7. Sister Jane Fell, *At Home in Many Worlds: Memoirs of an Iowa Farm Girl Who Had Far to Go* (Philadelphia: Medical Mission Sisters, 2011), 40.

8. Ibid.

9. Austin Moede, MD, telephone interview with the author, May 25, 2017.

10. Red Duke, interview by William H. Kellar, May 22, 2012.

11. Fell, *At Home in Many Worlds*, 44.

12. Ibid, 43.

13. Betty Duke Kent, interview by the author, June 9, 2016.

14. Ibid., January 8, 2016.

15. Ibid., telephone conversation with the author, December 12, 2016.

16. Dexter Filkins, "On Afghan Road, Scenes of Beauty and Death," *New York Times*, February 7, 2010.

17. Fell, *At Home in Many Worlds*, 44.

18. Ibid., 43.

19. Ibid., 44.

20. James P. Sterba, "In Kabul, Connally Meets His 1963 Dallas Doctor," *New York Times*, July 9, 1972.

Chapter 12

1. Bryant Boutwell and John P. McGovern, *Conversation with a Medical School: The University of Texas–Houston Medical School 1970–2000* (Houston: The University of Texas–Houston Health Science Center, 1999), 4.

2. Ibid.

3. Georgia Beth Johnson and Avrel Seale, "The Johnson Connection," *Texas Alcalde*, July 1997, 28, https://books.google.com/books?id=j84DAAAAMBAJ.

4. Mitchell Lerner, "Frank Craig Erwin, Jr. (1920–1980)," *The Handbook of Texas Online*, Texas State Historical Association, http://mcadams.posc.mu.edu/russ./testimony/shires.htm, https://tshaonline.org/handbook/online/articles/fer08.

5. Johnson and Seale, "The Johnson Connection."

6. Cheves McCord Smythe, *An Advantaged Life: Recollections of Cheves McCord Smythe, M.D.* (Atlanta: Team Forte, 2013), 354.

7. Ibid., 355.

8. Ibid., 354.

9. Ibid., 400.

10. Ibid.

11. William Henry Kellar and Heather Green Wooten, *Skilled Hands: Surgery at the University of Texas Medical School at Houston* (Houston: William Henry Kellar, 2016), 153.

12. Smythe, *An Advantaged Life*, 365.

13. Red Duke, interview by William H. Kellar, May 22, 2012.

14. Stanley Dudrick, email message to the author, December 19, 2016.

15. Kellar and Green Wooten, *Skilled Hands*, 34–35.

16. Red Duke, personal conversation with the author, October 24, 2014.

17. Ted Copeland, quoted in Kellar and Wooten, *Skilled Hands*, 36.

18. Red Duke, interview by the author, October 10, 2014.

Chapter 13

1. Steve Dunn, interview by the author, February 10, 2016.

2. Ibid.

3. "7 Cheat Death in Fiery Crash," *Abilene Reporter News*, March 4, 1963.

4. Steve Dunn, interview by the author, February 10, 2016.

5. Jan Jarboe Russell, "Flight for Your Life," *Texas Monthly*, March 1992, http://www.texasmonthly.com/articles/flight-for-your-life/.

6. Jules Vern, *Robur le Conquérant*, 1886, http://public.eblib.com/choice/public fullrecord.aspx?p=4719472.

7. "The History of the Air Ambulance," Angel MedFlight, blog, https://blog.angelmedflight.com/2014/01/14/the-history-of-the-air-ambulance/.

8. Richard DeLuca, "Igor Sikorsky and His Flying Machines," Connecticut History.org, http://connecticuthistory.org/igor-sikorsky-and-his-flying-machines/.

9. William G. Howard, "History of Aeromedical Evacuation in the Korean War and Vietnam War," thesis, US Army Command and General Staff College, Fort Leavenworth, Kansas, 2003.

10. *M*A*S*H*, 20th Century Fox Television, CBS, September 17, 1972– February 28, 1983.

11. Red Duke, personal conversation with the author, January 8, 2014.

12. "History of Air Ambulance and Medevac," Mercy Flight Western New York, accessed June 21, 2016, https://www.mercyflight.org/content/pages/medevac.

13. Ibid.

14. Coordinated Accident Rescue Endeavor, State of Mississippi: Project CARE-SOM, University of Michigan, digitized February 10, 2016.

15. Flight for Life, St. Anthony Health Foundation, https://www.stanthony healthfoundation.org/shf/programs/flight-for-life-colorado/.

16. Cheves McCord Smythe, *An Advantaged Life: Recollections of Cheves McCord Smythe, M.D.* (Atlanta: Team Forte, 2013), 404.

17. Red Duke, interview by the author, September 11, 2014. "Golden hour" discussion from a follow-up telephone conversation, September 14, 2014.

18. Dane Schiller, "Life Flight: Saving Lives for 40 Years," *Houston Chronicle*, August 17, 2016.

19. Red Duke, interview by the author, September 11, 2014.

20. Ibid., interview by William H. Kellar, June 5, 2012.

21. Ibid., interview by the author, September 11, 2014.

22. Ibid., interview by William Kellar, June 5, 2012.

23. Ibid., interview by the author, October 10, 2014.

24. Ibid., interview by William H. Kellar, June 5, 2012.

25. Ibid.

26. Bill Disessa, "October 23, 1989: Terror from Phillips Blast Still Haunts," *Houston Chronicle*, October 23, 1989.

27. Unidentified Life Flight pilot, personal conversation with the author, 1994.

28. "Memorial Hermann Life Flight's Advanced Capabilities," Life Flight, Red Duke Trauma Institute, http://trauma.memorialhermann.org/life-flight/capabilities/.

29. Russell, "Flight for Your Life."

30. Schiller, "Life Flight."

31. Red Duke, interview by the author, September 11, 2014.

32. Doggtyred, "In Memoriam, Hermann Hospital Life Flight 1," Pilots of America, July 17, 2010, https://www.pilotsofamerica.com/community/threads/in-memoriam-hermann-hospital-life-flight-1.36959/. No patient was on the helicopter at the time of the crash. This was a fueling run.

33. Schiller, "Life Flight."

34. Steve Dunn, interview by the author, February 10, 2016.

35. Red Duke, interview by the author, February 21, 2015.

36. Ibid.

37. "What Is a RAC?" Regional Advisory Councils, EMS Trauma Systems, Texas Department of State Health Services, https://www.dshs.texas.gov/emstraumasy stems/etrarac.shtm.

38. Russell, "Flight for Your Life."

39. *Accidental Death and Disability: The Neglected Disease of Modern Society*, prepared by the Committee on Trauma and Committee on Shock, Division of Medical Sciences, National Research Council, Washington, DC, September 1966.

Chapter 14

1. Harvey Grant Taylor, *Remembrances and Reflections* (Houston: UT Health Science Center, 1991), 167.

2. Ibid.

3. Ibid., 167–68.

4. Mark Carlton, interview by the author, December 7, 2014.

5. Ibid.

6. Ibid.

7. Ibid.

8. Production script, "Smoking, Additions and Health Consequences," *The Texas Health Report: A Syndicated Series of Health Related News Inserts with Dr. "Red" Duke*, August 1989. Writer/Producer Elaine Mays, Videographer Tom Eschbacher. This script is one of nearly three hundred scripts in Red Duke's files, each in a folder labeled with title and production dates. His initial handwritten draft in each folder is accompanied by a polished and typed production script formatted with video/chyron cues for the editor on the left and Red's narration on the right.

9. *Buck James*, TriStar Television, ABC, September 27, aired September 27, 1987–May 5, 1988, https://en.wikipedia.org/wiki/Buck_James.

10. Hank Duke, interview by the author, October 29, 1916.

11. Red Duke, interview by the author, September 17, 2014.

12. Susan Ayala, "'Cowboy Doc' Is an Unusual Candidate to Succeed Koop as Surgeon General," *Wall Street Journal*, June 6, 1989.

13. John Bryant, "Musical Medicine Man," *Austin American-Statesman*, June 26, 1986.

14. Tom Eschbacher, email message to the author, January 3, 2017.

15. "Our Reporter," as told by Tom Eschbacher in *Our Dr. Duke*, Rick Smith Gallery exhibit book honoring Dr. Red Duke, Memorial Hermann–Texas Medical Center Office of Public Affairs, August 2016.

16. Mark Carlton, interview by the author, December 7, 2014.

Chapter 15

1. Dee Brown, *Bury My Heart at Wounded Knee: An Indian History of the American West* (New York: Holt, Rinehart & Winston, 1970), Kindle edition, 265.

2. Ibid., 162.

3. Ibid., 336.

4. Ibid.

5. "Reverence for Life," Wikipedia, https://en.wikipedia.org/wiki/Reverence_for_Life.

6. Red Duke, acceptance remarks, Capstick Award 2015, Dallas Safari Club, Dallas, Texas, January 22, 2015.

7. Ibid., interview by the author, December 12, 2014.

8. William Souder, "100 Years after Her Death, Martha, the Last Passenger Pigeon, Still Resonates," *Smithsonian Magazine*, September 2014, http://www.smithsonianmag.com/smithsonian-institution/100-years-after-death-martha-last-passenger-pigeon-still-resonates-180952445/.

9. US Supreme Court, Martin v. Wadell, 41 US 16 Pet. 367 (1842), https://supreme.justia.com/cases/federal/us/41/367/case.html.

10. Douglas Brinkley, *The Wilderness Warrior: Theodore Roosevelt and the Crusade for America* (New York: Harper, 2009), 166.

11. "Theodore Roosevelt and Conservation," National Park Service, https://www.nps.gov/thro/learn/historyculture/theodore-roosevelt-and-conservation.htm.

12. Red Duke, interview by the author, September 17, 2014.

13. Jayar Daily, interview by the author, February 21, 2015.

14. Red Duke, interview by the author, February 21, 2015.

15. Cowan McTaggart, "Distribution and Variation in the Native Sheet of North America," *American Midland Naturalist* 24 (1940).

16. LaVan Martineau, *Rocks Begin to Speak* (Whittier, CA: KC Publications, 1976).

17. Red Duke, interview by the author, September 17, 2014.

18. Jack Ballard, *Bighorn Sheep* (Lanham, MD: Rowman & Littlefield, 2014), 72, https://books.google.com/books?id=SS4vBQAAQBAJ.

19. John Jefferson, "The Hanging of Red Duke," *Texas Parks and Wildlife Magazine*, October 8, 2016, http://tpwmagazine.com/archive/2016/oct/LLL_redduke/.

20. Red Duke, interview by the author, September 17, 2014.

21. Jefferson, "The Hanging of Red Duke."

22. Ibid.

23. Ibid.

24. Red Duke, interview by the author, September 17, 2014.

25. Jefferson, "The Hanging of Red Duke."

26. Red Duke, interview, September 17, 2014.

Chapter 16

1. Hallie Duke, email message to the author, January 18, 2017.

2. Ibid.

3. Rebecca Duke, email message to the author, January 19, 2017.

4. Ibid.

5. Red Duke, conversation with the author, September 11, 2014. Unlike her sisters' degrees, Rebecca's is in the fine arts, from the School of Visual Arts in New York City.

6. Charles King, interview by the author, October 29, 2016. This was a group interview with Hank Duke and his son Jesse; and Sara Duke, her son Waylon Roosma, and her husband Charles King.

7. Sara Duke, interview by the author, October 29, 2016.

8. Hank Duke, interview by the author, October 29, 2016.

9. Ibid.

10. Betty Duke Kent, interview by the author, January 8, 2016.

11. This was an observation made in the last entry of a travel journal that Red kept between June 23 and July 11, 1957.

12. Red Duke, interview by the author, December 12, 2014.

Chapter 17

1. Pam Duke Wisener, telephone interview by author, February 27, 2017. All quotations from Pam are from this interview.

2. Patty Read, interview by the author, October 18, 2016.

3. Red Duke, interview by the author, March 15, 2015.

4. Celeste Sheppard, email to the author, May 10, 2017.

5. Ibid., interview by the author, February 20, 2015.

6. Ibid.

7. Ibid., email to the author, May 10, 2017.

8. Ibid., interview by the author, February 20, 2015.

9. Ibid., email to the author, June 12, 2017.

10. Betty Duke Kent, telephone conversation with the author, December 14, 2016.

11. Ibid., interview by the author, January 8, 2016.

12. Ibid.

Chapter 18

1. *Our Dr. Duke*, Rick Smith Gallery exhibit book honoring Dr. Red Duke, Memorial Hermann–Texas Medical Center, August 2016. This small red book was produced by Memorial Hermann–Texas Medical Center Office of Public Affairs for a reception opening the *Our Dr. Duke* exhibit in the hospital's Rick Smith Gallery. Thirteen stories were selected for display in the exhibit and publication in the red book. Red's daughter, Sara, and her husband, Charles King, attended and provided personal remarks for the event.

2. "Our Healer," as told by T. "Cissy" Rivers in *Our Dr. Duke*.

3. "Our Minister," as told by Brijesh "Billy" Gill in *Our Dr. Duke*.

4. Joseph Love, email message to the author, December 13, 2016.

5. Ibid.

6. Giuseppe Colasurdo, personal conversation with the author, November 16, 2016.

7. "Our Servant," as told by Logan Rutherford in *Our Dr. Duke*.

8. Tom Flanagan remarks presented at Red Duke memorial service for Memorial Hermann–Texas Medical Center and UTHealth employees. Memorial Hermann–Texas Medical Center, Houston, Texas, September 2, 2015. These remarks were recorded and transcribed by the author and are located in Red Duke OPA files under "Interviews/Recordings." Tom Flanagan is VP and COO of Memorial Hermann–Texas Medical Center and was a longtime colleague of Dr. Duke on the Life Flight and hospital side.

9. Julia Q. Mitchell, personal conversation with the author relaying her late husband's story, April 21, 2016.

10. "Dr. James 'Red' Duke," written eulogy remarks by Jim Bertz, MD, DDS, presented at the family memorial service. Service held at the Jasek Chapel, Geo. H. Lewis & Sons, Houston, Texas, August 29, 2015.

11. Jim Bertz, telephone conversation with the author, November 29, 2016.

12. Ibid.

13. Ibid.

14. Red Duke, interview by the author, February 21, 2015.

15. Ibid., September 11, 2014.

16. Linda Mobley, interview by the author, October 18, 2016.

17. Red Duke, interview by the author, February 20, 2015.

18. Richard Andrassy remarks presented at Red Duke memorial service for Memorial Hermann–Texas Medical Center and UTHealth employees. Memorial Hermann–Texas Medical Center, Houston, Texas, September 2, 2015. When Dr. Andrassy (UTHealth chair of surgery) mentioned Red's innovations and sometimes unorthodox methodology, the surgeons and OR nurses and staff laughed and nodded in agreement, with one young surgeon shouting, "I had to go buy more brown sugar!" The spirit of the standing-room-only crowd approaching three hundred friends and colleagues was one of tears mixed with laughter.

19. Red Duke, interview by the author, September 11, 2014.

Chapter 19

1. Stanley Dudrick, interview by the author, December 29, 2014.

2. "Country Breakfast with Red Duke," *'Bout Time*, blog, October 31, 2014, http://www.uth.edu/blog/bout-time/.

3. *Albert Schweitzer*, directed by Jerome Hill, film, 1957, DVD, Roan Group, 2005.

4. Red Duke remarks, dedication of the Dr. James "Red" Duke Elementary School, Alvin Independent School District, Manvel, Texas, September 7, 2014. Transcript in possession of the author.

5. Betty Duke Kent, telephone conversation with the author, December 14, 2016.

6. Patty Read, interview by the author, October 18, 2016.

7. Betty Duke Kent, personal conversation with the author, February 25, 2016.

8. Linda Mobley, interview by the author, October 18, 2016.

9. Patricia Hipps, telephone conversation with the author, December 14, 2016.

10. Casey Slusher, interview by the author, April 7, 2016.

11. Hallie Duke, telephone conversation with the author, January 7, 2017.

A Note on Sources

Primary research materials came from the private collection of letters and photographs in the possession of Red's daughter, Sara Duke. Additional personal letters and photographs were made available by Betty Duke Kent. The remaining primary materials came from the University of Texas McGovern Medical School, the Memorial Hermann–Texas Medical Center, the John P. McGovern Historical Collections and Research Center, the University of Texas Southwestern Medical Center Health Sciences Digital Library and Learning Center, the Houston Metropolitan Research Center, and the Baylor University Texas Collection and University Archives in Waco, Texas.

Oral history interviews used in the preparation of the manuscript were conducted by the author from 2014 to 2016. Additionally, William H. Kellar conducted a series of interviews for the McGovern Medical School's surgery department's history, *Skilled Hands*, including interviews with Red Duke on May 22, June 5, July 17, and August 1, 2012.

Interviews Conducted by the Author

NAME	DATE OF INTERVIEW
James H. "Red" Duke Jr., MD	February 12, 2014 February 24, 2014 September 11, 2014 October 10, 2014 January 9, 2015 February 20, 2015 February 21, 2015 March 15, 2015
Betty Duke Kent	January 8, 2016 January 29, 2016 February 25, 2016 June 9, 2016

NAME	DATE OF INTERVIEW
Hank Duke	October 29, 2016
Rebecca Duke	November 4, 2016
Sara Duke, PhD	February 20, 2015 October 29, 2016
Hallie Duke, PhD	November 6, 2016
James Bertz, MD, DDS	February 21, 2015 November 29, 2016
Mark Carlton	December 7, 2014
Jayar Daily	February 21, 2015
Stanley J. Dudrick, MD	December 29, 2014
Steve Dunn	February 10, 2016
Linda Mobley, RN	October 18, 2016
Austin L. Moede, MD	May 5, 2017
Frank G. Moody, MD	January 28, 2015
Patty Read, RN	October 18, 2016
Celeste Sheppard, MD	February 20, 2015
Casey Slusher, PA	April 7, 2016
Pam Duke Wisener	February 27, 2017

Index